SEVEN
PILLARS
OF HEALTH

Also by Jay Solomon

Vegetarian Times' Vegetarian Entertaining

Great Bowls of Fire

Vegetarian Times' Low-Fat &
Fast Mexican Cooking

Lean Bean Cuisine

Vegetarian Rice Cuisine

Vegetarian Soup Cuisine

The Global Vegetarian:
Adventures in a Meatless Kitchen

A Taste of the Tropics

Global Grilling

Chutneys, Relishes, and Table Sauces

SEVEN PILLARS OF HEALTH

*Nutritional Secrets for
Good Health and Long Life*

JAY SOLOMON

PRIMA PUBLISHING

This book is not intended to replace medical guidance. Persons should consult their physicians before following any specific treatment or nutritional plan discussed in this book. Responsibility for any adverse effects resulting from the use of information in this book rests solely with the reader.

PRIMA PUBLISHING and colophon are registered trademarks of Prima Communications, Inc.

Library of Congress Cataloging-in-Publication Data

Solomon, Jay.
    Seven pillars of health: nutritional secrets for good health and long life / Jay Solomon.
      p.   cm.
    Includes bibliographical references and index.
    ISBN 0-7615-0862-7
1. Nutrition. 2. Health. I. Title.
RA784.S644 1997
613.2—dc21
                                                          97-1000
                                                           CIP

97 98 99 00 01 DD 10 9 8 7 6 5 4 3 2 1
Printed in the United States of America

HOW TO ORDER
Single copies may be ordered from Prima Publishing, P.O. Box 1260BK, Rocklin, CA 95677; telephone (916) 632-4400. Quantity discounts are also available. On your letterhead, include information concerning the intended use of the books and the number of books you wish to purchase.

Visit us online at http://www.primapublishing.com

*To Margaret Shalaby
and Richard and
Margaret Solomon*

Contents

Acknowledgments

THIS BOOK HAS ITS ROOTS IN A GUEST LECTURE I DELIV-
ered at Cornell University. Professor Mary Tabacchi invited me to
speak to her class titled "Nutrition and Wellness in the Resort,
Hotel, and Spa Industry." My lecture and cooking notes evolved
into the *Seven Pillars of Health*, an integrated and enlightened approach to healthy eating. With the help of Georgia Hughes and
Jennifer Fox of Prima Publishing, *Seven Pillars* made the giant leap
from ambitious vision to exciting reality.

During the course of researching this book, I had the good for-
tune to attend a series of vegetarian nutrition lectures offered by
Dr. T. Colin Campbell, professor of nutritional biochemistry at
Cornell. Dr. Campbell, a pioneer in the field of plant-based nutrition and diet, is also the director of the Cornell–China–Oxford
Project on Nutrition, Environment, and Health. Aside from offering a wellspring of insights into diet, health, and fitness, this
groundbreaking seminar was the first vegetarian nutrition class to
be offered at a mainstream university.

I would also like to thank Dr. Banoo Parpia, senior research as-
sociate of the Cornell–China–Oxford Project, for generously shar-
ing her expertise about the virtues of a diversified plant-based
diet. In addition, I would like to thank Theresa Lyczko, M.S. CHES,

for allowing me to tap into her experiences as the health education director of the Healthy Heart Program of Tompkins County in New York.

Several agencies and institutions provided valuable nutritional data and advice, including the American Heart Association, National Cancer Institute, American Cancer Society, American Institute for Cancer Research, Center for Science in the Public Interest, American Dietetic Association, and Cornell Cooperative Extension.

Finally, I would like to thank again my "kitchen cabinet" of unofficial advisors: Shaun Buckley, Robert and Amy Cima, Sarah Huber, Leslie Goodyear, Marilee and Eamonn Murphy, Fredrica Pollack, Jessica Robin, the Robin Family, Beth Ryan, and Leslie Sadoff. My immediate family members—Jesse, Ann, Greg, Lisa, and my grandmother Mary Solomon—all contributed their distinct perspectives on the challenges of eating well and maintaining a healthy lifestyle. Of course, I owe a tremendous debt of gratitude to my wife, Emily, who has been with me since Day One—and has enthusiastically tasted every recipe in this book.

Introduction

THE QUEST FOR A HEALTHY LIFE BEGINS IN THE KITCHEN. The food we eat has the potential to promote better health, provide energy and sustenance, offer protection against a host of chronic diseases, and slow down the rate of aging. Healthy food offers nourishment, renewal, and enrichment—all while pleasing the palate and satisfying the appetite. A good diet forms the cornerstone of a vibrant and rewarding lifestyle.

Seven Pillars of Health is an enlightened guide to nutritious eating. Here are the essential principles and virtues of the healthy diet, from antioxidants, fiber, plant proteins, and complex carbohydrates to lowfat, low-cholesterol cuisine, the secrets of cooking with fire and spice, and phytochemicals, the "phytomins" of the future. Each pillar is illustrated with a cornucopia of worldly recipes, kitchen secrets, and good-for-you cooking tips. This is a comprehensive and integrated approach to eating well and living better.

Seven Pillars of Health bridges the gap between the plethora of up-to-date nutritional advice and the enticing world of gourmet cookery. The nutritional information presented is based on the very latest research and revelations. The recipes and cooking advice are gleaned from a culinary career spanning over twenty years in the professional kitchen. The principles of healthy eating are augmented with high-spirited, easy-to-understand recipes. From savory soups and succulent salads to hearty main courses, bold side dishes, refreshing sauces, and tempting desserts, here is vivid proof that healthy food can be both *nutritious* and *delicious*. *Seven Pillars* is a call for celebration, not deprivation.

While most people are vaguely aware of the basics of good nutrition, the path to optimum wellness is hobbled with detours and forks in the road. There are right turns and wrong turns, good choices and bad choices. The "right foods"—vegetables, fruits, grains, beans, starches—provide valuable antioxidants, fiber, vitamins, and phytonutrients. A diet rich in the right foods can be a potent weapon against chronic disease, fatigue, and aging. On the other hand, a poor diet weighed down with the wrong stuff—saturated fats, refined sugars, excess calories, and salt—can wreak havoc on one's health and well-being.

Unfortunately, many of us travel down the wrong path far too often. The typical American meat-and-potatoes diet is fat-laden, turbo-caloried, super salty, and sometimes syrupy sweet. Most diets are notoriously lacking in the health-enhancing nutrients, fiber, energy, and protective substances found in plant foods. Many of us also tend to indulge until we are stuffed, pause a few minutes, then attack dessert. Snacking and nibbling are ongoing pursuits with no distinct beginning, middle, or ending. That eating is a national pastime is not the problem; we simply eat too much of the wrong kind of foods.

Not surprising, over two-thirds of Americans are overweight—and many are tipping the scales toward obesity. Despite the proliferation of health clubs, exercise videos, and high-tech sneakers, the collective girth of the country is expanding, not shrinking. Somewhere along the line, life has become an "all-you-can-eat" buffet. On the flip side, fewer than ten percent of the general public consumes the recommended "five-a-day" servings of fruits and vegetables. Furthermore, a glaring minority of people consume the proper amount of fiber, complex carbohydrates, and plant-based nutrients.

Of course everyone wants to look and feel healthy. However, a combination of confusion, misunderstanding, and everyday temptations have collectively thwarted the best of intentions. Advice often appears contradictory: one day, margarine is said to be better than butter; the next day, the reverse is true. Oat bran is "in," then "out," then "in" again. Sound bites about health and diet all seem to blur and morph together. Understandably, it is hard to make sense of the mayhem and keep up with the abundance of breakthroughs that flood the media on a daily basis.

Beleaguered by the cacophony of advice, many people simply tune out and fill up (with second helpings). Others appease their conscience by popping vitamin pills on the way to raiding the refrigerator. To the chagrin of nutritionists, the nemesis of the healthy diet—hot dogs, hamburgers, chicken nuggets, and sausages—are considered standard fare on the American table. Food choices are too often based on convenience and haste, not healthfulness or taste.

In the quest for a healthy life *Seven Pillars of Health* offers a ray of hope. This book enthusiastically encourages the shift from the typical animal-based, high-fat diet to a plant-based diet rich in vegetables, fruits, grains, starches, and legumes. This is not a radical notion; the vast community of doctors, nutritionists, and health officials routinely urge the public to *decrease* their intake of fatty foods, red meat, processed meals, and salty junk food and to *increase* their consumption of fresh vegetables, whole grains, beans, fruits, and starchy foods. *Seven Pillars* simply provides the tools—the three R's, so to speak—to make the change: Rationale, Recipes, and Resolve. (After tasting the recipes, the resolve comes easy.)

There is overwhelming evidence that a well-balanced, plant-based diet rich in vegetables, fruits, grains, and legumes can promote good health, offer protection against disease, and replenish the body with energy and vitality. Based upon this bedrock premise, the seven pillars form the foundation of a healthful diet. When complemented with a healthy lifestyle, the seven pillars might even help you build your body into a temple of good health and well-being.

Seven Pillars of Health depends on synergy—every pillar holds an important place on the path to wellness. There are no miracle pills or single ingredients that promise to cure society of its ailments. To focus on only one nutrient is akin to judging a city's skyline by staring at one solitary building. *Variety* and *diversity* are the keys to a healthy diet. The best way to keep the doctor away is to eat an apple a day, as well as an orange and banana, and tomorrow try a star fruit and mango, then maybe a tangerine or pineapple. The virtues of a plant-based diet come to fruition when a wide range of fruits and vegetables are consumed. Variety is not only the spice of life, it is the linchpin of a healthy diet.

Here is an overview of the *Seven Pillars of Health*.

Pillar 1: Unleash the Power of Antioxidants

Antioxidants are a diverse family of nutrients and enzymes found in colorful plant foods such as leafy greens, oranges, winter squash, tomatoes, and tropical fruits. Whole foods rich in antioxidants may play a significant role in preventing heart disease, certain cancers, premature aging, and other chronic diseases. Antioxidants have the potential to become the "super vitamins" of tomorrow.

The antioxidant family includes vitamin C, vitamin E, lycopene, selenium, and carotenoids such as beta-carotene and lutein. These antioxidants may prevent disease by protecting our bodies against oxidation, a natural "rusting" process. Oxidation is accelerated by scavenger "free radicals" roaming in our bodies; the SWAT team of antioxidants attack and neutralize the harmful free radicals. In doing so, antioxidants obstruct the oxidation process and help to reduce the occurrence of cell damage and disease. (When cells are damaged, a window of opportunity is open for disease.)

An ounce of antioxidant prevention may be worth a pound of cure. This pillar of health features a glossary of good food sources for antioxidant nutrients, such as butternut squash, pumpkin, citrus fruits, kale, tomatoes, mangoes, broccoli, and whole grains. To help boost your intake of antioxidants, there is an array of antioxidant-rich recipes to choose from, including Pumpkin Rice and Red Beans, Lemon-Braised Market Greens with Sunflower Seeds, Portuguese Greens Soup, Pasta with Tomato-Carrot Ragu, and Pumpkin-Molasses Muffins.

Pillar 2: Discover the Goodness of Fiber

Fiber comes with an impressive résumé of health benefits. Also called roughage, fiber refers to the chewy, indigestible parts of vegetables, fruits, beans, and other plant foods. Fiber-rich foods can promote regularity, relieve constipation, and help to prevent a host of chronic diseases such as colon cancer, heart disease, and obesity. The inconvenient "everyday ailments" that plague so many Americans (such as irregularity) can often be relieved by switching to a high-fiber diet.

This pillar explores the virtues of two primary groups of dietary fiber, *soluble* and *insoluble*, and features ways to include fiber-rich foods as part of a healthy diet. From beans, apples, cruciferous vegetables, and bananas to leafy greens, potatoes, whole grains, and bran cereals, there is a cornucopia of good-for-you foods sated with fiber. There is also a wide assortment of fiber-rich recipes to pique your palate, including Garden Three-Bean Salad, Country Black Bean Soup, White Bean and Corn Chili, and Banana-Blueberry Bran Bread.

Pillar 3: Treasures of the Heart: Secrets of Lowfat, Low-Cholesterol Cooking

Most everyone is vaguely familiar with the double trouble associated with dietary fat and cholesterol. There is a mountain of evidence linking high-fat, high-cholesterol diets to an increased risk of heart disease, stroke, obesity, and other ailments. To health officials, fat and cholesterol are Public Enemies Number One and Two.

Familiarity does not always breed understanding. This pillar of health untangles the web of good and bad cholesterol, healthy and unhealthy fats, and deciphers the role of trans-fatty acids, fake fat, and body fat. If this sounds daunting, do not despair; it is possible (and easy) to reduce the fat and cholesterol in one's diet without resorting to radical measures. In this war against fat, your taste buds (as well as your health) will declare victory.

Furthermore, lowfat cookery does not have to be bland, uninspired, or a synonym for abstinence or austerity. To the contrary, this pillar of health proves that lowfat, heart-smart cookery can be bold and adventurous. The contingent of high-flavored recipes will transform the notion of humdrum lowfat cooking into a delicious art form. The menu of recipes includes Orange-Zucchini Muffins, Kiwi Vinaigrette, Penne Pasta with Lemony Swiss Chard, and Creole Vegetable Hot Pot. With a pantry filled with indispensable staples such as olive oil, canola oil, wine vinegars, flavored liquids, and citrus fruits, there is a profusion of flavor in the lowfat kitchen (but little fat and cholesterol!).

Pillar 4: Exploding the Protein Myths

Protein is a nutrient with a false halo over its head. This is an important (but often overrated) nutrient. The average diet contains twice as much protein as the recommended daily allowance. The popular penchant for protein comes with a price tag; recent research has established a possible link between diets rich in animal-based protein (such as red meat and poultry) with heart disease, stroke, hypertension, and other ailments. In addition, animal protein travels with saturated fat and cholesterol, two other villains of the healthy diet. Most animal foods are concentrated sources of protein and fat and conspicuously lack antioxidants, phytochemicals, fiber, and complex carbohydrates.

On the other hand, despite what many believe, the protein derived from a plant-based diet of vegetables, grains, and legumes can supply more than an ample amount of our daily needs. The vegetable proteins synthesized from beans, rice, grains, soy foods, and other plant foods come with negligible fat and cholesterol and travel with "the good stuff"—antioxidants, phytochemicals, fiber, and essential vitamins. Although by themselves plant foods offer "incomplete" proteins, it is easy to form complete proteins within the context of a well-balanced diet.

There are multiple myths connected with protein; this pillar of health confronts the maze of beliefs (and misbeliefs) head-on. In addition to examining the myths, the pillar also deciphers the nature of amino acids, the building blocks of protein. There is an expansive glossary that includes ways to cook with protein-rich plant foods, such as beans, lentils, quinoa, amaranth, tofu, and soy milk. The roster of balanced-protein recipes includes Super Grain Cornbread, Red Bean Ratatouille Stew, Black Bean Succotash, and Blueberry-Banana Soy Shake.

Pillar 5: Fire and Spice: High-Flavor, Low-Sodium Cooking with Herbs, Spices, and Chili Peppers

In the pursuit of intense flavors with minimal salt, enter the trio of herbs, spices, and chili peppers. These assertive seasonings play a central role in today's heart-healthy cookery and liven up meals in ways that a salt shaker could only dream of. From pungent cilantro, refreshing mint, and earthy thyme to sweet nutmeg, aromatic allspice, and searing Scotch bonnet peppers, this pillar covers the gamut of exciting flavors and powerful aromas.

The problem is that Americans love salt. Moderation is a fine concept, but the average diet contains *ten* times the recommended daily allowance of sodium (a component of salt). Sodium can be found everywhere, from processed foods (canned vegetables), cured meats, and snack foods to commercial breads, dressings, and condiments. A high sodium intake has been linked to hypertension (high blood pressure), a cardinal risk factor for heart disease and stroke. While the sodium-hypertension link is generally ignored by the public, as people grow older blood pressures are sure to rise. Sodium is one factor that should not be dismissed lightly.

Salt cheats the taste buds from experiencing more invigorating and diverse flavors. This pillar of health offers an extensive glossary on the anti-salt brigade: garden herbs, dried herbs, and fragrant spices (and spice blends); there is also a complete guide to cooking with a variety of hot chili peppers. With a little fire and spice in the kitchen, there is little need for cream, butter, and salt—the triple threats to the healthy diet. This pillar also features a range of highly spiced recipes that will wake up your palate, from Garden Herb Pesto and Yellow Spice Rice to Curried Squash with Chick-Peas and Jamaican Jerk Vegetables.

Pillar 6: Power Eating with Complex Carbohydrates: Boosting Energy with Rice, Grains, Pastas, and Potatoes

Complex carbohydrates form the centerpiece of a healthful diet. The carbohydrate "power foods"—whole grains, brown rice, pasta, beans, yams, and fruits—provide our bodies with long-lasting energy and stamina. Carbohydrate-rich foods satisfy our appetite, dilute the desire to overeat, and come with an enriching package of essential vitamins, minerals, and beneficial fiber.

There are two basic kinds of carbohydrates: complex carbohydrates (also called starches) and simple carbohydrates (also called sugars). Although both types are converted into glucose, our body's unit of fuel, complex carbohydrates (potatoes and grains) provide high-octane fuel, whereas simple sugars (candy bars and refined foods) provide cheap fuel that burns off quickly, zaps our energy, and fades away. The difference between complex carbohydrates and simple sugars is the difference between lightning and a lightning bug, to paraphrase Mark Twain.

This pillar of health offers appealing dishes fortified with power foods: wheat, barley, quinoa, wild rice, legumes, pastas, potatoes, and a variety of rices. From Power Chowder, Wild Rice and Split Pea Soup, and Gourmet Spaghetti with Braised Greens to Powerhouse Pilaf and Farmers' Market Risotto, the recipes promise to be hearty, flavorful, and brimming with nutrients.

Pillar 7: On the Trail of Phytochemicals: Vitamins of the Future

For years nutritionists have asserted that a diet rich in vegetables, fruits, grains, and legumes can reduce the risk of certain cancers, heart disease, and other chronic illnesses. Recently scientists have discovered the specific compounds in plant foods that attack or obstruct the inner core of disease at the cellular level. This family of natural plant substances is called "phytochemicals" (*phyto* comes from the Greek word for plant).

Specifically, there are hundreds of phytochemicals that can potentially ward off or wipe out cancerous cells at several different stages of development. Although these "phytomins" have tongue-twisting names (such as isoflavones, sulforaphane, and genistein), they are making the world sit up and take notice. Just as the discovery of vitamins a century ago helped to wipe out scurvy, pellagra, and other diseases, phytochemicals may help win the battle against the modern era of chronic degenerative diseases. Phytochemicals could be the future of disease prevention.

Like the family of antioxidants, phytochemicals serve as important signposts along the journey to a healthy life. This pillar of health features an easy-to-understand reference for phytochemicals as well as a glossary of widely available phytochemical-rich foods, such as cabbage, broccoli, onions, soy foods, tomatoes, and berries. The menu of alluring phyto-friendly recipes includes Hot Cabbage Gumbo, Onion Pumpkin Bread with Sunflower Seeds, and Leafy Turnip Tureen.

In the pursuit of health and happiness there are numerous factors in life that we cannot control. The air we breath, the water we drink, our family history, the environment, and the invisible hand of fate all influence our long-term health and well-being. But there is one major factor we can assert control over: the food we eat. Diet plays a critical role in the quality of everyone's life. Choose a healthy diet, and you choose to live a better and more fruitful life.

The seven pillars form the building blocks of a healthy diet. This book cuts a swath through the forest of information and blazes a road to health and wellness. *Seven Pillars of Health* is a beacon of optimism and offers hope that eating right today will lead to a better and healthier tomorrow.

—Jay Solomon

SEVEN
PILLARS
OF HEALTH

Pillar 1

UNLEASH THE POWER OF ANTIOXIDANTS

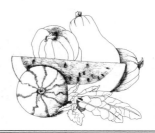

Our parents were right after all: fruits and vegetables really are good for us. As we head into the twenty-first century, it has become clear that the merits of plant foods are far greater than ever imagined. There is a mountain of evidence to suggest that a plant-based diet can decrease the risks of cancer, heart disease, cataracts, and other chronic diseases of the Western world. It turns out that an apple a day really *will* keep the doctor away—if it comes with a diet loaded with beans, whole grains, sturdy vegetables, dark leafy greens, and colorful fruits.

Nutritionists and researchers are discovering that people who eat plenty of fruits and vegetables also tend to lead healthier, longer, and more fruitful lives (no pun intended). The big question is, why? There is more than one answer to this complex issue, but widespread attention is shifting to a family of nutrients and enzymes called *antioxidants*. Whole foods rich in antioxidants may help prevent chronic illnesses and premature aging. Simply put, antioxidants help our bodies fight off disease.

By preventing and protecting our bodies against long-term disease (and sometimes reversing the damage), antioxidants play a

1

major role in the pursuit of a good and healthy life. As Ben Franklin once said, an ounce of prevention is worth a pound of cure. Put another way, more trips to the greengrocer may cut back on future trips to the pharmacy.

The diverse family of antioxidants includes vitamin C, vitamin E, lycopene, selenium, and carotenoids such as beta-carotene and lutein. Most of these antioxidants are found naturally in a variety of plant foods. Not all antioxidants are vitamins in the traditional sense of the word. Some antioxidants are the color pigments in plants, while other substances are minerals or naturally occurring plant chemicals. For example, the antioxidant lycopene puts the red in tomatoes, while beta-carotene gives carrots, sweet potatoes, and winter squash their orange and yellow hues.

Antioxidants may be the super nutrients of tomorrow. About a century ago the discovery of vitamins led to the conquering of scurvy, pellagra, rickets, and other diseases. Unfortunately, vitamins did not cure every problem. Modern civilization is afflicted by other scourges. Heart disease, cancer, stroke, and cataracts affect millions of people every year. In this new era of age-related (lifestyle) diseases, a "SWAT team" of plant-based antioxidants is leading the charge against disease.

There is still much to be learned about antioxidants. Research will continue to yield new breakthroughs, and most likely there will be even more antioxidants detected and identified in the future. However, one thing seems certain: a burgeoning corps of antioxidants can promote health, prevent illness, and assist in the ongoing quest for a good and healthy life.

UNDERSTANDING THE POTENTIAL OF ANTIOXIDANTS

How do antioxidants work? There is strong reason to believe that antioxidants strike at the roots of disease itself, down at the cellular level. Antioxidants appear to help prevent healthy cells from becoming damaged. When cells are damaged, deteriorate, or become *oxidized,* the stage is set for a variety of diseases to develop (such as heart disease or cancer). In fact, a process called oxidation is one of the major factors in cell damage and related diseases.

A preponderance of research suggests that a diet high in antioxidant-rich foods can help safeguard our bodies against the dangers of harmful oxidation.

To thoroughly understand the power of antioxidants, one must first grasp the dual concepts of oxidation and free radicals. Oxidation is a kind of natural and gradual "rusting" process happening in cells all the time, all day, every day. The process is similar to the browning of a sliced apple or a stick of butter turning rancid. This oxidation process can be accelerated by several environmental factors such as cigarette smoking, too much sunlight, pollution, and exposure to harmful chemicals and toxins in foods.

The process of oxidation is interrelated with *free radicals,* a group of highly reactive particles that roam and rampage about within our bodies. Free radicals are the chief suspects in accelerating the oxidation process. Additionally, free radicals have been accused of "crimes" against our health. Free radicals may speed up the aging process, increase the levels of artery-clogging "bad" cholesterol in our bodies, attack DNA, and conspire to cause damage to healthy cells. In short, free radicals advance the progress of disease by adding gasoline to the fire.

Scientists are quick to point out that not all free radicals are evil; in fact, some are necessary for fighting harmful cells. Oxidation is necessary for life to exist, but too much oxidation (and too many free radicals) is not a good thing. More often the free radicals in our bodies are on a mission to attack, invade, and destroy healthy cells and make the body vulnerable to disease. Remember, when healthy cells deteriorate, the door is opened to disease. Too many free radicals can endanger our well being.

Unfortunately, oxidation, free radicals, and toxins are a part of everyday life. We are exposed to all kinds of toxins—in the air we breathe, the foods we eat, the liquids we drink. Some toxins are even produced naturally in our bodies. To achieve good health (and to *feel* healthy), the challenge is to ward off and thwart as

A preponderance of research suggests that a diet high in antioxidant-rich foods can help safeguard our bodies against the dangers of harmful oxidation.

many free radicals as possible. That's where antioxidants enter the equation: by attacking and arresting free radicals, antioxidants prevent cells from being damaged, sweep away harmful toxins, and in the process, help protect against disease.

A WALK ON THE BRIGHT SIDE: ANTIOXIDANTS TO THE RESCUE

Antioxidants are the valiant bodyguards against scavenging free radicals and help us avoid and limit destruction wrought by oxidation. Experts believe that antioxidants tie up and neutralize the free radical "pirates" before they can wreak havoc. In the process, antioxidants help prevent cell damage and disease from occurring. By disarming, attacking, and tying up free radicals, antioxidants can prevent the inception of a variety of free radical–related diseases including cancer, arteriosclerosis, and cataracts. There is even proof that antioxidants may slow down the normal aging process. By nipping so many potential problems in the bud, antioxidants keep the fountain of youth flowing.

In a nutshell: a diet loaded with antioxidant-rich fruits and vegetables can help prevent the oxidation process from ripping apart cells and savaging our bodies. Fruits and vegetables are not only good for us (as our parents had insisted) but may also help protect us from debilitating chronic diseases and premature aging. A plant-based diet consisting of antioxidant-rich carrots, winter squash, dark leafy greens, tomatoes, and oranges may provide the best insurance against long-term disease and the best chance for lasting health.

THERE ARE NO MAGIC BULLETS, BUT . . .

Granted, there are many factors involved in the goal to achieving optimum health and well-being. Other considerations include alcohol consumption, smoking habits, family and personal history, and environmental factors. For example, it has been estimated that bad habits and an unhealthy way of life are responsible for 65 percent of cancer deaths. Think of it: the chance to live a healthy, disease-free life may rest, at least partially, in the food we choose to eat over the course of our lifetime.

Food, more than fate, determines our destiny. Choosing to eat a variety of nutrient-dense, antioxidant-rich fruits and vegetables is the first step to achieving a healthier and more fruitful life, and to decreasing the risk of chronic degenerative diseases.

ANTIOXIDANTS: AN IN-DEPTH LOOK

There are five well-known antioxidants that have shown promise in fighting disease and preserving health. Keep in mind that the best research suggests that antioxidants are interdependent and work as a team, not as individual units. The best way to derive their benefits is not to focus on one or two antioxidants, but to eat a plant-based diet comprising a variety of whole foods. When it comes to the family of antioxidants, the whole is greater than the sum of the parts.

Vitamin C: The Super Vitamin

Vitamin C is perhaps the most famous antioxidant and has been hailed as a cure for everything from the common cold to cancer. Also called *ascorbic acid*, vitamin C performs myriad tasks such as helping to heal wounds, maintaining connective tissue (collagen), facilitating iron absorption, enhancing the immune system, and fortifying the body's resistance to infection and colds. (*Ascorbic* comes from the Latin *ascorbutus*, "without scurvy.")

Scientifically speaking, as a water-soluble antioxidant vitamin C offers the first line of defense against free radicals in the blood plasma surrounding the cells. It seems that vitamin C neutralizes

Food, more than fate, determines our destiny. Choosing to eat a variety of nutrient-dense, antioxidant-rich fruits and vegetables is the first step to achieving a healthier and more fruitful life, and to decreasing the risk of chronic degenerative diseases.

the free radicals before they can attack our cell membranes. In addition, vitamin C also has a synergistic relationship with vitamin E. In a sort of tag-team defense, when vitamin E expends itself after a reaction with free radicals, vitamin C is able to recycle vitamin E back to normal. Additionally, studies have linked high intake of vitamin C with a decreased risk of developing several cancers including stomach, lung, oral, and liver cancers.

There is an ongoing debate about the effects of taking megadoses of vitamin C in the form of supplements. A well-balanced diet of fruits and vegetables can deliver 200 milligrams of vitamin C (the optimal daily level recommended by most nutrition experts). Excessive amounts of vitamin C obtained from vitamin pills (some contain 1,000 milligrams) are excreted by the body, not absorbed.

To fully benefit from vitamin C's antioxidant powers, head to the produce section of the grocery store, not the pharmacy aisles. Nature has provided a bounty of whole foods teeming with vitamin C.

How to Eat More Vitamin C–Rich Foods

Citrus fruits are the obvious choices: oranges, tangerines, and grapefruits make healthful snacks any time of day. Tangy lemons and limes can bring flavor to rice dishes, leafy greens, salads, and soups. Other good sources include potatoes, spinach, collards, broccoli, cantaloupe, red peppers, berries, and tropical fruits.

For a quick hit of vitamin C, peel a kiwi or eat a wedge of cantaloupe for a snack; pack a peach or nectarine for lunch; cook with red peppers (both sweet and hot varieties contain vitamin C); squeeze fresh lemon over braised spinach or salad greens (the vitamin helps the body absorb iron); baste corn on the cob with lime instead of butter; drink orange juice, not iced tea; add fresh berries to breakfast cereal.

Freezing does not drastically reduce the vitamin C content. However, cooking, canning, and long-term storage do reduce the vitamin amount. For best results, use quick cooking methods such as stir-frying, blanching, and steaming. Also, prepare dishes that retain the cooking liquid (such as pilafs, risotto, and soup meals). For optimal flavor, purchase fresh fruits and vegetables close to the time of consumption, not in large, economy-size batches. Make a point to visit the local greengrocer on a frequent basis.

Beta-Carotene, Lutein, and the Carotenoids

There are over five hundred plant-based carotenoids, including beta-carotene, lutein, and alpha-carotene. Carotenoids are prevalent in orange, yellow, and dark green vegetables and fruits such as carrots, winter squash, and spinach (the chlorophyll in green plants hides the orange pigment). Butternut squash, sweet potatoes, mangoes, apricots, cantaloupe, canned and fresh pumpkin, and mesclun greens are additional food sources of carotenoids. (See Table 1.1.)

Beta-carotene is the most abundant carotenoid and has also received the most attention by researchers and the media. As a precursor to vitamin A, beta-carotene is converted by the body into the vitamin after it is digested and absorbed. For years, beta-carotene was valued primarily as a building block for vitamin A, an essential nutrient. To date, there is no RDA for beta-carotene.

The public spotlight shifted to beta-carotene after numerous studies revealed that diets high in beta-carotene–rich fruits and vegetables led to a decreased risk of heart disease and certain cancers. In fact, there have been hundreds of studies linking high blood levels of beta-carotene with reduced risk of several diseases. Beta-carotene is believed to neutralize unstable free radicals and inhibit the growth of cancerous cells. When the news got out, a range of food products from bran cereal to margarine began touting the addition of beta-carotene as a health claim.

Of course, beta-carotene's bubble was about to burst. A Finnish study reported that when heavy, long-term smokers were given doses of beta-carotene supplements, they experienced a slightly higher rate of lung cancer. The widely publicized study garnered headlines and cast a pall over beta-carotene. Skeptics of healthful eating had yet another reason to ignore or scoff at dietary edicts.

But it is important to read between the headlines. First of all, the study was conducted with middle-aged Finnish men who had been smoking for over thirty years and maintained questionable dietary practices. No vitamin supplement is going to reverse a life-time of unhealthy habits. Second, beta-carotene was consumed in the form of supplements, not derived from whole foods. Third, the study had little relevancy to nonsmokers.

If anything, the Finnish results proved that when beta-carotene is isolated, the antioxidant benefits may be nullified. However—and this is a big however—the results do not contradict the hundreds of studies that have linked beta-carotene–rich foods with preventative (i.e., antioxidant) powers against disease. This is one more reason to focus on eating nutrient-dense whole foods rather than vitamin supplements, and to scrutinize any health discoveries reported on the evening news.

Research continues to evolve. It is most likely that beta-carotene teams up with other carotenoids, such as alpha-carotene; antioxidants; or phytochemicals to prevent disease and promote good health. If anything, beta-carotene is a nutrient marker for other protective substances in fruits and vegetables that help our bodies defend against disease.

In an effort to learn more about other carotenoids, researchers are targeting beta-carotene's less hyped cousins that are also found in yellow, orange, and green plant foods. For example, *lutein* and *zeaxanthin* found in kale, broccoli, chard, and mustard greens have been shown to offer protection against age-related macular degeneration—a common cause of blindness among the elderly. Alpha-carotene, another carotenoid in carrots, may bolster the immune system. More studies are underway, so stay tuned for future news on carotenoids. In the meantime, fill your plate with carotenoid-rich fruits and vegetables.

How to Eat More Carotenoid-Rich Foods

Add diced carrots to soups, green salads, and stews; roast winter squash or sweet potato for a side dish; blend mashed pumpkin

TABLE 1.1

Antioxidant Friendly Carotenoids

Carotenoid	Plant Sources
Alpha-Carotene	Canned and fresh pumpkin and carrots
Lutein and Zeaxanthin	Broccoli, kale, spinach, chard, mustard greens, and turnip greens
Beta-Cryptoxanthin	Mangoes, papayas, oranges, and tangerines

into soups, muffins, and breads; lightly braise dark green leafy vegetables (such as kale, spinach, or chard) with lemon or wine; add sweet potatoes to potato salad, chowder, pilafs, or mashed vegetable dishes; pack a few wedges of cantaloupe or papaya for lunch; peel a mango for dessert; combine peaches, mango, and berries with soy milk for a fruity shake.

Vitamin E: The Heart-Smart Nutrient

Vitamin E, also called *tocopherol*, has been hailed as a white knight against heart disease. There is strong reason to believe that vitamin E prevents bad cholesterol from building up in arteries (evidently it prevents the oxidation of cholesterol, a factor leading to plaque buildup). By reducing cholesterol's ability to gum up arteries, vitamin E plays a significant role in preventing a heart attack or stroke. Additionally, vitamin E protects cells from the potential dangers wreaked by highly reactive free radicals. High doses of vitamin E have also been credited with reducing the occurrence of blood clots and with enhancing immune functions.

Vitamin E is a fat-soluble nutrient, and it is the one antioxidant that is difficult to consume in large amounts strictly from whole foods—and without piling on the fat. It is prevalent in unprocessed vegetable oils such as canola oil, sunflower oil, and corn oil, as well as in food products made with vegetable oils such as margarine and mayonnaise. (That doesn't mean load up on the mayonnaise or margarine—they are loaded with fat!) Additional sources of vitamin E include wheat germ, whole grain cereals, nuts, seeds, legumes, asparagus, avocados, sweet potatoes, spinach, and leafy greens. Since many sources of vitamin E are high in fat, health experts universally agree that in this isolated case, taking vitamin supplements might not be such a bad idea, albeit in the context of a well-balanced, healthy diet.

How to Eat More Vitamin E–Rich Foods

Sprinkle hazelnuts or almonds over a green salad; add sunflower seeds to muffins and breads; add wheat germ to breakfast cereals, fruit shakes, and baked goods; use unprocessed vegetable oils for cooking, baking, and salad dressings; add a sliced avocado to your sandwich in place of cold cuts; roast a sweet potato; eat whole grain cereals.

Lycopene: The Red Antioxidant

The news media have widely reported the health-enhancing potential of *lycopene*, a recently recognized antioxidant. Why? One study concluded that men who regularly consumed tomatoes and tomato-based dishes such as pizza, pasta with red sauce, tomato soup, and other tomato dishes were associated with a reduced rate of prostate cancer. Lycopene, a carotenoid that gives tomatoes their red pigment, has since been ordained as a key antioxidant offering protection against not only prostate cancer but also colon and bladder cancer.

The ruby red carotenoid is found in fresh tomatoes and the plethora of canned tomato products including tomatoes that have been sauced, juiced, stewed, puréed, and crushed. This is a rare case in which canning actually concentrates (rather than reduces) the amount of nutrients available. Lycopene is also present in watermelon, pink grapefruit, and guava.

How to Eat More Lycopene-Rich Foods

Serve pasta dishes with meatless red sauces, marinara sauce, or raw tomato sauces (and avoid high-fat cream sauces); choose tomato salsa over sour cream dips or cheese dips; eat tomato-based dishes such as Creole sauce, pasta with arrabbiata (spicy red sauce), ratatouille, and tomato-based soups; order traditional pizzas with tomato sauce, not trendy white pizzas; and eat pink grapefruits, not white grapefruits.

Selenium: The Antioxidant Mineral

Touted as an anti-aging weapon, *selenium* works with vitamin E to maintain normal cell metabolism and promotes skin elasticity (i.e., prevents wrinkles). Other studies have tied selenium with reducing the risk of several types of cancer, curbing the spread of destructive viruses, and bolstering the immune system by helping the body produce crucial antioxidant enzymes.

Selenium can be found in nuts (especially unshelled Brazil nuts), whole grains (oats, brown rice, wheat bran), sunflower seeds, seafood, and garlic. The mineral is especially abundant in grains and vegetables grown in selenium-rich soil.

How to Eat More Selenium-Rich Foods

Add chopped unsalted cashews to a garden salad, stir-fry, or chili; sprinkle unprocessed bran or wheat germ over breakfast cereals; eat multigrain breads made with oatmeal, nuts, and/or seeds; snack on uncracked nuts.

THINK OF ANTIOXIDANTS AS NATURE'S RAINBOW FOODS

To maximize the benefits gained from antioxidants, fill your plate with a variety of antioxidant-rich "rainbow foods" all year long. From salsa and tomato sauce to brown rice pilaf, squash risotto,

TABLE 1.2

The Family of Antioxidants: Tomorrow's Super Nutrients

Antioxidant	Plant Sources (and Shopping List)	Characteristics
Vitamin C	Citrus fruits, broccoli, cantaloupe, kiwi, mangoes, dark leafy greens, tomatoes, berries, cabbage, red peppers, and cranberries	The first line in defense against free radicals. Enhances immune system; facilitates the absorption of iron in leafy greens.
Vitamin E	Wheat germ, nuts, seeds, whole grain cereals and breads, and vegetable oils	Credited with preventing "bad" cholesterol from clogging arteries.
Beta-Carotene (precursor to vitamin A)	Carrots, sweet potatoes, winter squash, pumpkin, dark leafy greens, mangoes, papayas, cantaloupe, apricots, peaches, and nectarines	Present in orange, yellow, and dark green plant foods (green chlorophyll hides the pigment).
Lycopene	Tomatoes and tomato products (juiced, stewed, puréed, and crushed), watermelon, and pink grapefruit	Prostate protector; abundant in tomatoes and canned tomato products. (Lycopene is not affected by the heating process.)
Selenium	Whole grains, nuts (Brazil nuts, cashews), and sunflower seeds	Grains grown in selenium-rich soil are good sources. Uncracked nuts appear to be a better source than salted, processed nuts.

braised greens, and hearty tomato-vegetable soups, there is a bounty of savory heart-healthy meals to choose from. In addition, your consumption of antioxidant-rich foods will ensure that you also benefit from the contingent of disease-fighting fiber, phytochemicals, and vitamins found in plant foods (see Table 1.2). In the process, you'll also reduce your intake of saturated fat, cholesterol, and fatty calories—the enemies of the healthful lifestyle.

On the other hand, you won't find many antioxidants present in fast-food restaurant fare, snack foods, deli meats, or animal-based foods. Neither steaks nor hamburgers nor turkey breasts nor chicken pot pie offer much in the way of antioxidants.

To fully exploit the healing powers of antioxidants, the meat portion of a meal must be moved to the side or completely off the plate. Vegetables, grains, and starches must be moved to the center of the plate.

THE ADVANTAGES OF EATING WHOLE FOODS (VERSUS POPPING A PILL)

It should come as no surprise that many people would prefer to gulp a super antioxidant pill than to maintain a nutritious well-balanced diet. It might be easier to swallow a capsule and call it a day, but the culinary rewards of healthy eating would be missed. Besides, it has not yet been proven whether antioxidants in supplement form can deliver the same protective, life-enhancing benefits derived from whole foods. Research on antioxidant supplements have delivered mixed and muddled results. When it comes to the merits of supplements, the jury is still debating the issue.

What's wrong with supplements? Experts believe that antioxidants work in synergy with each other and with other micronutrients that have not yet been identified. Synthetic pills have yet to replicate the healing potential of whole foods. The family of carotenoids, vitamins, minerals, and phytochemicals perform complementary roles within our bodies, assist each other in the battle against disease, and network with hundreds of other beneficial substances. When antioxidants are isolated and consumed as supplements, a decreased level of preventative activity has been observed. Nature seems to be saying: get your antioxidants from the garden, not from a capsule.

To fully exploit the healing powers of antioxidants, the meat portion of a meal must be moved to the side or completely off the plate. Vegetables, grains, and starches must be moved to the center of the plate.

There is a saying in sports, "the best offense is a good defense." When it comes to the game of healthy living, a plant-based diet teeming with antioxidant-rich vegetables and fruits offers the best defense against the opponent of the good life, namely, chronic degenerative disease. In sports, a good defense can win games. In the real world, eating with a smart game plan can pave the way to a healthier and more rewarding life.

Granted, there is still much to be learned about the role of antioxidants in disease prevention and how the various nutrients work in synergy with each other. However, the bottom line remains clear: to reap the benefits of antioxidants, eat a variety of rainbow foods: vegetables, fruits, whole grains, and legumes. And while there are plenty of sound nutritional reasons to *eat your spinach,* the recipes contained throughout this book should provide plenty of epicurean enticements as well.

When it comes to the game of healthy living, a plant-based diet teeming with antioxidant-rich vegetables and fruits offers the best defense against the opponent of the good life, namely, chronic degenerative disease.

TEN EASY WAYS TO EAT MORE ANTIOXIDANT-RICH FOODS

1. Include dark leafy greens in salads and avoid nutrient-weak iceberg lettuce.
2. Snack on exotic tropical fruits (such as mangoes, papayas, star fruit, and kiwi).
3. Add diced tomatoes to condiments such as pesto, salsa, guacamole, and black bean dip.
4. Choose tomato-based dishes such as chili, red sauce for pasta, and tomato-vegetable soup.
5. Pack a fruit snack for lunch (peaches, oranges, nectarines, and/or apricots).
6. Buy a "juicer" (a juice extractor) or blender designed for processing vegetable and fruit shakes.
7. Add diced sweet potatoes or winter squash to soups and rice dishes.
8. Cook with whole grains such as wild rice, brown rice, or bulgur.

9. When traveling, seek out vegetarian options on restaurant menus.
10. Eat vegetarian dinners three or four times a week.

ANTIOXIDANTS IN THE KITCHEN

Carrots

Carrots are one of the most nutritious and versatile vegetables. The crunchy orange roots are loaded with beta-carotene, soluble fiber, vitamin C, and other carotenoid pigments. (Come to think of it, carotenoids derived their name from carrots.) If carrots are not a regular staple on your shopping list, then you are not eating enough of them.

Shredded carrots make a colorful salad garnish; carrot sticks and baby carrots make a healthful snack and are perfect for dipping into hummus, guacamole, and bean dips. Cooked carrots add flair to soups, pilafs, stews, tomato sauces, muffins, pancakes, and sweet breads. When combined with apples, celery, parsley, and cabbage, carrots form the basis of a delicious and nutrient-dense fresh juice.

Dark Leafy Greens

Dark leafy greens include a cornucopia of leaf lettuces, green and red vegetable leaves, mustards, and cabbages. Some greens are the edible tops of root vegetables (i.e., turnip greens and beet greens); others are stalklike, tightly furled bunches (red and green chard, kale, and bok choy); still others are feathery and fernlike (dandelion greens, frisee, and mizuna). Some varieties should be cooked first, while others can be eaten raw. Dark leafy greens are versatile, easy to prepare, highly nutritious, and widely available throughout the year.

The beauty of cooking with greens is that most are interchangeable and blend well with each other. For instance, mild red chard can be combined with assertive kale or turnip greens; bok choy blends well with Chinese cabbage and mizuna; broccoli rabe is leavened with red Russian kale. Mixing and matching brings out well-rounded flavors and textures.

Leafy greens are good sources of vitamin C, carotenoids, fiber, phytochemicals, iron, folacin, and calcium. (Chlorophyll, a green pigment, overshadows the beta-carotene's orange tint.) Generally speaking, the darker the leaf, the more nutritious and flavorful the dish. Green leaf lettuce and Romaine lettuce contain far more nutrients than pale iceberg lettuce, which is rather weak in the nutrient department. (By now most health-conscious people are aware that iceberg is a poor excuse for a lettuce.)

Here are a few general tips for preparing leafy greens at home.

Selection: Look for leafy greens free of tears, yellow spots, and blemishes. A healthy bunch of greens should be trimmed of any damaged leaves. As a general rule, smaller leaves are usually more tender and succulent.

Storage: Wrap unwashed greens in a moistened paper towel and place the bunch in a plastic bag, then refrigerate. Leave the bag partially open to allow for air flow. Most greens will keep for five to seven days.

Preparation: Pluck out any wilted or discolored leaves and remove the thick fibrous parts of the stems. Place the greens in a colander and immerse in a cold bath of water (such as a vegetable sink or large bowl). Swish the greens around and let sit for a minute; the sand and debris should drift to the bottom. (Some greens can be placed in a colander and rinsed under cold running water.) Drain the colander and shake off any excess liquid, or use a salad spinner. After the greens are washed and cleaned they are ready to be coarsely chopped or cut into ribbonlike strips (*chiffonade-style*).

Cooking Tips: Braising is a healthy way to cook leafy greens. Braising refers to cooking the greens in a small amount of liquid—either water, citrus juice, wine, or vegetable broth. Braised greens can include aromatic ingredients such as garlic, onions, white beans, chili peppers, tomatoes, and balsamic vinegar. Greens can also be steamed, microwaved, or blanched (briefly boiled) like other green vegetables.

Soup Greens: When used as a vegetable, leafy greens add contrasting colors and flavors to simmering soups and stews such as minestrone, potato chowder, black bean soup, curried bisques, tomato-based broths, and other hearty tureens. Simply chop and stir the greens into the pot about ten to fifteen minutes before the finish. Some greens (such as collards and turnip greens) hold up well in slow-cooked soups. Adding greens to a soup is also a way to maximize nutrient retention—the cooking liquid doubles as the broth.

One-Pot Dishes: Leafy greens can also be added to pilafs, risotto, stews, and one-pot grain dishes. Coarsely chop the greens and stir into the pot ten to fifteen minutes before the finish. Greens add character to red sauces for pasta, lasagna, pasta primavera, stir-fries, and sautéed dishes. As with soups, adding greens to a pilaf or one-pot dish maximizes nutrient retention since the cooking liquid is absorbed by the rice, grain, or sauce.

Salad Greens: There is a multitude of leafy greens that add zesty flavors to tossed green salads. Although sturdy varieties of greens are ideally cooked first, some varieties such as chard, bok choy, and beet greens can be eaten raw if they are young and tender. (For a glossary of salad greens, see page 118.)

A Cook's Guide to Leafy Greens

Here is a glossary of popular leafy greens found in the healthful kitchen. Unless otherwise noted, most of these greens are available in well-stocked supermarkets, natural food stores, or ethnic markets.

Amaranth, also called red sen choy, has large green leaves marked with striking reddish purple streaks. Amaranth tastes similar to spinach. The young leaves can be added raw to salads, and the larger leaves can be cooked like spinach. The greens are available in Asian markets, natural food stores, and farmers' markets.

Beet Greens are the leafy tops attached to beet roots. They are similar to red chard in appearance and exhibit a mustardy, radishlike flavor. (Chard is actually a member of the beet family.) Young beet greens can be added raw to salads, while larger greens can be blended into cooked dishes.

Bok Choy Greens are tall, floppy dark leaves with crisp, white stems. Bok choy has a mild cabbage flavor and collardlike texture. The leaves are typically cut into ribbonlike strips before cooking. Two similar greens, *tat soi* and *pat soi* (also called baby bok choy), have smaller, more tender leaves and make colorful additions to tossed salads.

Broccoli Rabe, also called rapini or broccoli raab, resembles a leafy bouquet of budding miniature broccoli florets. A favorite green in Italian and Asian cooking, broccoli rabe has an assertive, mustardy flavor (some regard it as a bitter taste). Broccoli rabe is often sautéed with garlic and olive oil and served with risotto or pasta.

Chard, also known as Swiss chard, really refers to two varieties, red chard and green chard. Red chard leaves have beet-colored veins, while green chard have thin, white veins. (There is a lesser-known deep purple variety that can turn a dish pink.) Chard greens have a crunchy texture and a mild mustard flavor. (Chard is a member of the beet root family.) Young chard leaves can be added raw to tossed salads.

Collards are a well-known staple of the Southern kitchen. Collard greens are large, sturdy, deep green leaves that are flat, not curled. The cruciferous vegetable tastes like a cross between kale and cabbage. The greens can be braised, boiled, or added to long-cooking soups and stews. Collards take about 20 minutes to cook, although traditional recipes may call for longer times.

Escarole is a mildly flavored leafy vegetable popular in Italian cuisine. The wide, furled, green leaves look somewhat like a green iceberg lettuce. Escarole can be braised with garlic, wine, and olive oil or added to soups and pasta dishes.

Frisee is a feathery, mild leaf with an apple-green hue and jagged leaves. Also called French chicory, frisee has a faintly bitter taste. It is often blended into mesclun salads or served with a warm dressing. A quick braising brings out its subtle mustard flavor.

Kale is an overlooked and underrated leafy vegetable. The crinkled, pale olive green leaves have a mild cabbage and spinach flavor and firm texture. The loose leaves make a nutritious addition to soups and stews. (Kale inspired the classic *caldo verde,* a Portuguese soup.) Kale can be braised, stir-fried, and added to pilafs and red sauces. Don't miss out on this healthful leafy green.

Mizuna is a narrow, fernlike green with a slight peppery flavor (similar to arugula). Popular in Japanese cooking, mizuna can be braised, steamed, or tossed raw into a salad. Mizuna is available in Asian markets and natural food stores.

Red Russian Kale, a close cousin of kale, has flat, purplish green leaves with a serrated oak leaf–like shape. Russian kale has limited availability but is a farmers' market favorite and is worth the hunt. It can be added to soups, stews, and one-pot dishes. The young leaves can be tossed into leafy salads.

Do not confuse red Russian kale with salad savoy (also known as flowering kale or purple kale). Salad savoy has a tightly bunched head and comes in shades of white, green, and purple. The colorful leaves are bitter, coarse, and better suited for garnishing, not eating.

Southern Greens loosely refers to mustard greens, dandelion greens, and turnip greens. This family of greens is distinguished for its sharp mustardy flavors and bitter nuances. The sturdy, versatile greens can be added to soups, stews, and rice or pasta dishes. Southern greens can also be braised or steamed for a healthy side dish.

Spinach is perhaps the most popular leafy green. It can be eaten raw or cooked and is absolutely packed with nutrients. When raw, the crisp leaves perk up salads and sandwiches; when braised or sautéed, the flavor becomes concentrated and the leaves lose much of their bulk. Spinach adds life to lentil and bean stews, tossed pasta salads, soups, grain dishes, red sauces, and many other dishes. In addition to antioxidants, spinach contributes protein, folacin, calcium, and iron. (Citrusy fruits can facilitate the iron absorption.)

Sweet Potatoes

Sweet potatoes are close cousins to white potatoes but are from a completely different plant family—they are roots, not tubers (like potatoes). The naturally lowfat, sweet, orange flesh is rich in beta-carotene, vitamin C, and complex carbohydrates, and the skin contains fiber. Sweet potatoes should not be limited to the holiday table; like white potatoes, they can be mashed, roasted, grilled, and added to salads, soups, stews, and grain dishes. (They make a great substitute for white potatoes in vichyssoise.)

Tomatoes

Tomatoes are luscious red fruits that are eaten like vegetables. Tomatoes have inspired a multitude of dishes, from pizza, salsa, and pasta with red sauce to vegetable juice, Italian soups, Indian curries, Creole dishes, and spicy stews. The red pigment in tomatoes—lycopene—has been associated with reduced occurrence of prostate cancer. Tomatoes also contain vitamin C, beta-carotene, and numerous phytochemicals, including p-coumaric acid and chlorogenic acid.

Garden tomatoes are great for salads, salsa, sandwiches, and uncooked sauces. The brigade of canned tomato products—stewed, crushed, puréed, whole, diced, and so forth—are indispensable staples in the healthful pantry. Canned tomato products make excellent sauces, soups, chili, and stews. Recently a variety of enticing designer tomatoes (with names like "brandy wine," "purple cherokee," "sun gold," and "evergreen") have appeared at the greengrocer, but the best tomatoes tend to be the old-fashioned varieties grown in the backyard.

Tropical Fruits

Tropical fruits are loaded with vitamin C, fiber, potassium, and other essential nutrients. Not too long ago tropical fruits were scarce and expensive, but today's markets have expanded the selection and availability. Kiwi fruits, for example, were once considered exotic but are now as familiar as apples and bananas.

Tropical fruits can be sliced and diced and added to fruit salads or green salads; packed as a snack; combined into dressings, salsas, and chutneys; blended into desserts; or added to fresh juices and shakes. They add a taste of pizzazz to the meal.

A Cook's Guide to Tropical Fruits

Here is a glossary of popular tropical fruits. Unless otherwise noted, most of these fruits are available in well-stocked supermarkets, natural food stores, or ethnic markets.

Citrus Fruits are edible powerhouses of vitamin C. The contingent includes oranges, tangerines, grapefruits, ugly fruits (a cross between a grapefruit and an orange), limes, lemons, mandarins, and blood oranges. A freshly peeled citrus fruit makes a wonderful afternoon snack.

Kiwi Fruit is the little, brown, oval fruit with a green flesh and endearing sweet-and-tart flavor, a cross between a strawberry and a banana. Kiwi fruits were once a specialty of New Zealand, but most of today's fruits are California-grown and widely available throughout the year. Kiwi fruits can be added to fresh juice, salad dressing, and fruit salads. Peel and eat for a light snack.

Mango is the quintessential tropical fruit. The taste invokes flavors of pineapple, citrus, and nectarine. Mangoes tend to have a kidney shape and green skin marked with reddish orange hues. The coral-orange flesh is rich in beta-carotene, vitamin C, and fiber. Like an avocado, a ripe mango should give a little when pressed. (Green, unripe mangoes have a crunchy, raw potato–like texture and less desirable bland taste.)

To prepare a mango, peel its skin like a potato and cut the flesh off the rather large pit. Add the vibrant coral-orange flesh to fruit salad, a soy milkshake, fresh juice, fruit chutney, salad dressings, or salsa. Buy two and eat one out of hand. You won't regret trying one.

Papaya is a pale green fruit with a mild, cantaloupelike flavor. Although some papayas grow as large as a watermelon, most are the size of a miniature football. The fruit contains the enzyme *papain,* which aids in digestion, as well as fiber, carotenoids, and loads of vitamin C. To eat, scoop out the inner black seeds, and then scoop out the coral flesh.

Pineapple, the royalty of tropical fruits, has a citrusy-sweet aroma when ripe. To buy a ripe pineapple, look for one with a yellowish brown skin and a distinctive tropical aroma. A ripe pineapple should give slightly when pressed with your fingertips. Diced pineapple can be added to fruit salads and juice, baked goods, chutneys, and dressings.

Star Fruit, also called carambola, is a sweet-and-tart citrusy fruit with fantastic thirst-quenching qualities. When a star fruit is sliced crosswise, the slice resembles a star, hence the name. The greenish yellow fruits are tart, but the bright yellow fruits are ripe and sweet. The whole fruit is edible, even the few seeds. Just rinse, slice, and enjoy.

Winter Squash

Winter squash come in a motley variety of shapes, sizes, and colors. Despite their name, winter squash are available throughout most of the year. (They are also called hard-shelled squash.) Winter squash are versatile, easy to prepare, and interchangeable in most recipes.

The sturdy gourds are good sources of beta-carotene, vitamin C, potassium, and fiber. Squash with deep orange flesh have more beta-carotene than pale orange varieties. Winter squash are also low in calories, sodium, and fat.

Here are tips to buying, storing, and preparing the hefty gourds.

Selection: When choosing a winter squash, look for hard, firm shells free of blemishes, soft spots, or broken skins. The stems should be still attached. Pick up and hold the squash; it should feel heavy and dense.

Storage: Winter squash will keep for several months if kept in a cool, dark place and away from oven heat or sunlight. Peeled and diced squash can be refrigerated for several days or frozen.

Preparation: To roast a large round squash, cut the gourd in half with a sharp knife and remove the seeds and stringy fiber. Place the squash in a baking pan filled with about 1/4-inch water; roast in a preheated 375-degree F oven until the pulp is easily pierced with a fork, about 30 to 40 minutes.

Butternut squash is the easiest squash to peel and dice for soups and one-pot dishes. Cut off the bell-shaped bottom and the stem. Stand the tubelike part of the squash on a cutting board and with a knife (or vegetable peeler) cut down on the squash and remove the thin layer of skin. Cut the squash lengthwise into celerylike strips, then dice. (Some supermarkets now carry pre-peeled butternut squash.)

A Cook's Guide to Winter Squash

Unless otherwise noted, most winter squash are available in well-stocked supermarkets, natural food stores, or ethnic markets. Peak season is from late summer to early winter.

Acorn squash are shaped like a large acorn with pleated ridges. The dark green gourds are naturally decorated with sporadic streaks of golden orange and yellow. Easy to roast, acorn's flesh is mild and soft.

Blue Hubbard is so large that it is often sold in wedges. It has a pale bluish gray skin and a surprisingly vibrant orange flesh. Blue Hubbard tastes somewhat like butternut squash or West Indian pumpkin.

Buttercup squash are dark green gourds with portly, rotund shapes. The bronze-orange flesh is mildly sweet and buttery and can be roasted like acorn squash.

Butternut are the most versatile winter squash and are widely available. The squash have long, tan necks and bell-shaped, bulbous ends where seeds are stored. The orange flesh has a sweet potato–like sweetness and melds easily into soups, grain and rice dishes, risotto, and sauces. Simply peel, dice, and add to the pot.

Delicata are sometimes called sweet potato squash. They have a sweet, yellowish orange flesh and are treasured for their buttery flavors. The small, elongated squash have ribbed skins and green, white, or orange streaks. Roasted delicata usually makes one serving.

Kabocha are cherished in Japanese cuisine. The rotund, dark green gourds have a dense orange flesh and sweet-and-savory taste. Kabocha can be roasted like acorn squash.

Pumpkin refers to two main varieties: small sugar pie and large field pumpkins ("jack-o-lanterns"). Sugar pie pumpkins have a dense, rich flesh and are commonly used for cooking. Field pumpkins are mildly flavored, seedy, and often used as Halloween ornaments. For convenience, canned pumpkin is a good kitchen staple (and contains a concentrated amount of beta-carotene).

Red Kuri squash, also called Golden Hubbard, is a large, reddish orange squash with a thin skin and delectable flesh. Similar in flavor to Blue Hubbard and West Indian pumpkin, red kuri is a farmers' market staple and is widely available in autumn. A squash connoisseur's favorite.

Sugar Loaf and *Sweet Dumpling* are small, sweet-tasting squash similar to the delicata in flavor. The squash are interchangeable with delicata and acorn squash and can be roasted and served as a single serving.

West Indian Pumpkin, also called calabaza, is a huge, gigantic gourd with a bold orange, sweet-tasting flesh. The skin varies from tan and orange to streaky forest green. The shape can be round like sugar pie pumpkin or elongated and heavy like a watermelon. West Indian pumpkin is often sold in pre-cut wedges in Caribbean and Hispanic markets. It is occasionally available in well-stocked supermarkets or natural food stores.

SIGNATURE RECIPES FOR THE ANTIOXIDANT-RICH, HEALTHY DIET

Mango-Papaya Vinaigrette

Super Carotenoid Cocktail

Curried Squash Bisque

Beta "Carrotene" Bisque

Sweet Potato Vichyssoise

Portuguese Greens Soup

Gazpacho with Bulgur

Wintry Squash Risotto

Pumpkin Rice and Red Beans

Sweet Potato Pilaf with Brown Rice

Savory Squash Pilaf

Italian-Braised Rapini with Tomatoes

Lemon-Braised Market Greens with Sunflower Seeds

Tuscan Greens and White Beans

Wine-Braised Kale with Wild Mushrooms

Native Squash and Hominy Stew

Gourmet Squash with Maple Syrup

Pasta with Tomato-Carrot Ragu

Pumpkin-Molasses Muffins

Additional health benefits are noted with each recipe.

Mango-Papaya Vinaigrette

This ultra-nutritious dressing endows a green salad with a touch of tropical flair. The riper the fruit, the sweeter the dressing.

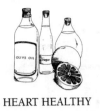

HEART HEALTHY

1 large mango, peeled, pitted, and diced
1 large papaya, peeled, seeded, and diced
1/3 cup canola oil
1/4 cup apple cider vinegar
1 tablespoon honey
1/2 teaspoon white pepper
1/4 teaspoon salt

Place all of the ingredients in a food processor fitted with a steel blade or in a blender and process for about 10 seconds until smooth. Pour into a serving container. Drizzle the dressing over tossed green salads. Refrigerate the remaining dressing for later.

YIELD: ABOUT 2 CUPS (12 TO 14 SERVINGS)

Super Carotenoid Cocktail

HEART HEALTHY

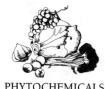

FIRE AND SPICE

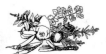

PHYTOCHEMICALS

Drinking a glass of fresh juice is an easy and efficient way to load up on antioxidants. The juice also happens to be brimming with refreshing flavors.

4 medium carrots, peeled
2 large red apples, cored and cut into wedges
4 to 6 large leaves kale or chard
1 large stalk celery
$1/2$ cup parsley leaves
$1/2$ lemon or lime, peeled and quartered
1 small wedge of beet root (optional)

Place all of the ingredients, piece by piece, into a juice extractor while it is running. Stir the fresh juice, pour into glasses, and serve. For extra fiber, stir a few tablespoons of the pulp into the juice.

YIELD: 2 SERVINGS

Curried Squash Bisque

Curry provides an aromatic and pungent flavor to this smooth vegetable bisque. Squash melds mellifluously into the soup broth.

HEART HEALTHY

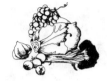

PHYTOCHEMICALS

2 teaspoons canola oil
1 large yellow onion, diced
1 cup sliced celery
2 large tomatoes, diced
3 to 4 cloves garlic, minced
2 teaspoons minced fresh ginger
2 to 3 teaspoons curry powder
2 teaspoons ground cumin
1¹/₂ teaspoons dried thyme
1 teaspoon salt
¹/₂ teaspoon black pepper
4 cups peeled, diced butternut or other winter squash
2 cups coarsely chopped spinach or kale
¹/₄ cup chopped fresh parsley

In a large saucepan heat the oil over medium heat. Add the onion and celery and cook, stirring, for about 5 minutes. Add the tomatoes, garlic, and ginger and cook, stirring, for 3 to 4 minutes more. Stir in the curry powder, cumin, thyme, salt, and pepper and cook for 1 minute more over low heat, stirring frequently. Add the squash and 5 cups of water and bring to a simmer. Cook for about 20 minutes over medium-low heat until the squash is tender. Stir in the greens and parsley and cook for 5 to 10 minutes more over low heat.

Transfer the soup mixture to a food processor fitted with a steel blade or to a blender and process for 5 to 10 seconds until smooth. Pour the soup into serving bowls and serve hot.

YIELD: 6 SERVINGS

Beta "Carrotene" Bisque

This soup combines carrots and sweet potatoes—two carotenoid-rich vegetables—into one delicious soup.

HEART HEALTHY

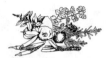

FIRE AND SPICE

1 tablespoon canola oil
1 medium yellow onion, diced
1 large stalk celery, chopped
2 cloves garlic, minced
4 cups water or vegetable broth
2 cups diced sweet potatoes
1 cup diced carrots
1 teaspoon ground coriander or cumin
$1/2$ teaspoon salt
$1/2$ teaspoon black pepper
$1/2$ teaspoon curry powder or turmeric
1 cup lowfat milk or soy milk
2 tablespoons chopped fresh chives or parsley (for garnishing)

In a large saucepan heat the oil over medium heat. Add the onion, celery, and garlic and cook, stirring, for 5 minutes. Add the water, sweet potatoes, carrots, coriander or cumin, salt, pepper, and curry powder or turmeric and bring to a simmer. Cook over medium-low heat for 20 to 25 minutes, stirring occasionally, until the vegetables are tender.

Remove the soup from the heat and transfer to a blender or food processor fitted with a steel blade. Purée for about 5 seconds until smooth. Return the soup to the pan and stir in the milk. (Gently reheat if necessary.) Ladle into bowls and sprinkle the herbs over the top before serving.

YIELD: 4 SERVINGS

Sweet Potato Vichyssoise

This healthful spin on traditional potato and leek soup offers a savory way to highlight carotenoid-rich sweet potatoes in a meal.

HEART HEALTHY

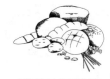

POWER EATING

1   tablespoon canola oil
1   medium yellow onion, diced
2   cups chopped leeks, rinsed
2   large cloves garlic, minced
4   cups water or vegetable stock
4   cups peeled, coarsely chopped sweet potatoes
2   medium carrots, diced
1/4 cup dry white wine
1/2 teaspoon salt
1/2 teaspoon white pepper
3   tablespoons chopped fresh parsley
1   to 2 tablespoons chopped fresh dill
1   cup lowfat milk or soy milk

In a large saucepan heat the oil over medium heat. Add the onion, leeks, and garlic and cook, stirring, for about 5 minutes. Add the water or stock, sweet potatoes, carrots, wine, salt, and pepper and bring to a simmer. Cook over medium-low heat for about 25 minutes, stirring occasionally. Stir in the parsley and dill and let cool for about 5 minutes.

Transfer the soup to a blender or food processor fitted with a steel blade and purée for about 5 seconds until smooth. Return the soup to the pan and stir in the milk. Return the soup to a gentle simmer. Ladle into warm bowls and garnish with extra sprigs of herbs.

YIELD: 6 SERVINGS

Portuguese Greens Soup

Known as "caldo verde," this wholesome soup is filled with potatoes, kale, and white beans.

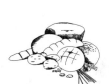

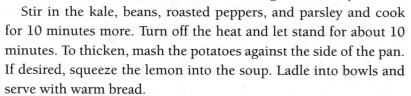

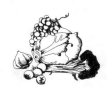

1 tablespoon olive oil
1 medium yellow onion, diced
2 or 3 large cloves garlic, minced
4 cups diced white potatoes (peeled if desired)
1/2 teaspoon salt
1/2 teaspoon white pepper
2 cups chopped, packed kale
1 can (15 ounces) white kidney beans, drained
1/4 cup diced roasted sweet red peppers
1/4 cup chopped fresh parsley
1 large lemon, quartered (optional)

In a large saucepan heat the oil over medium heat. Add the onion and garlic and cook, stirring, for 4 minutes. Add 4 cups water, potatoes, salt, and pepper and bring to a simmer. Cook for about 20 minutes over medium heat, stirring occasionally.

Stir in the kale, beans, roasted peppers, and parsley and cook for 10 minutes more. Turn off the heat and let stand for about 10 minutes. To thicken, mash the potatoes against the side of the pan. If desired, squeeze the lemon into the soup. Ladle into bowls and serve with warm bread.

YIELD: 6 SERVINGS

Gazpacho with Bulgur

This chilled summer soup boasts the nutrients of a liquid salad. Grains of bulgur add sustenance and texture.

HEART HEALTHY

POWER EATING

- ½ cup bulgur
- ¾ cup boiling water
- 2 large ripe tomatoes, diced
- 1 small red onion, diced
- 1 medium red bell pepper, seeded and diced
- 1 medium cucumber, peeled and diced
- 1 small jalapeño pepper, seeded and minced
- 2 cloves garlic, minced
- ¼ cup chopped fresh parsley
- 3 to 4 tablespoons chopped fresh basil
- 1 teaspoon Tabasco or other bottled hot sauce
- 1 teaspoon ground cumin
- ¼ teaspoon black pepper
- ¼ teaspoon salt
- 2 cups canned tomato juice (preferably low sodium)

In a small saucepan or bowl combine the bulgur and boiling water. Cover and set aside for 15 minutes.

In a large mixing bowl combine the remaining ingredients. Place three-quarters of the mixture in a blender or food processor fitted with a steel blade and process for 5 seconds, forming a vegetable mash. Return to the bowl and blend with the remaining vegetables and bulgur. Chill for 30 minutes to 1 hour before serving.

Ladle the gazpacho into chilled bowls and serve with French or Italian bread.

YIELD: 4 TO 6 SERVINGS

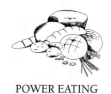

Wintry Squash Risotto

Cooked winter squash melds seamlessly into this creamy dish of Italian risotto.

$1^1/_2$ tablespoons olive oil
8 ounces button mushrooms, sliced
1 medium yellow onion, finely chopped
3 or 4 cloves garlic, minced
2 cups peeled, diced butternut squash or red kuri squash
$1^1/_2$ cups arborio rice
1 large carrot, diced
$^1/_2$ teaspoon white pepper
$^1/_2$ teaspoon salt
$^1/_2$ teaspoon turmeric
1 cup green peas, fresh or frozen
$^1/_3$ to $^1/_2$ cup grated Parmesan cheese

In a large saucepan heat the oil over medium heat. Add the mushrooms, onion, and garlic and cook, stirring, for about 5 to 6 minutes. Stir in 3 cups water, the squash, rice, carrot, pepper, salt, and turmeric. Cook (uncovered) over medium heat for about 10 minutes, stirring frequently.

Gradually stir in another 2 cups water and the peas and cook for 12 to 15 minutes more, continuing to stir, until the rice and squash are tender.

Remove from the heat and fold in the cheese. Let stand for about 5 minutes before serving. Serve with warm bread.

YIELD: 4 SERVINGS

Pumpkin Rice and Red Beans

This festive dish is traditionally made with West Indian pumpkin, a huge squash with a vibrant, sweet potato–like flesh. Butternut or red kuri squash can be substituted.

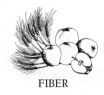

FIBER

1 tablespoon canola oil
1 medium yellow onion, chopped
2 large cloves garlic, minced
2 cups peeled, diced West Indian pumpkin or butternut squash
2 teaspoons curry powder
1/2 teaspoon black pepper
1/2 teaspoon salt
1/4 teaspoon ground cloves
1 1/2 cups white rice (try basmati)
1 cup coarsely chopped kale or spinach
1 can (15 ounces) red kidney beans, drained

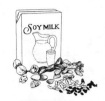

PROTEIN

POWER EATING

In a large saucepan heat the oil over medium heat. Add the onion and garlic and cook, stirring, for 5 minutes until the onion is translucent. Stir in the pumpkin, curry, pepper, salt, and cloves and cook for 1 minute more.

Add 3 cups water and the rice, cover, and bring to a simmer. Cook over medium-low heat for about 15 minutes. Stir in the kale and beans and cook for about 5 minutes more. Fluff the rice and turn off the heat. Let stand for 10 to 15 minutes before serving.

YIELD: 4 TO 6 SERVINGS

HELPFUL HINT

Serving rice and beans with chicken or fish is a great way to elevate the nutrients of the meal.

Sweet Potato Pilaf with Brown Rice

HEART HEALTHY

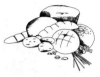

POWER EATING

Adding sweet potatoes to a simmering pilaf is a quick and easy way to include carotene-rich vegetables in a meal.

1 tablespoon canola oil
1 medium yellow onion, diced
8 to 10 button mushrooms, chopped
2 cloves garlic, minced (optional)
1 medium sweet potato, scrubbed and diced
1 cup long grain brown rice
$^1/_2$ cup orzo
$^1/_2$ teaspoon salt
$^1/_2$ teaspoon black pepper
$^1/_2$ teaspoon ground turmeric or curry powder
2 whole scallions, chopped

In a saucepan heat the oil over medium heat. Add the onion, mushrooms, and garlic and cook, stirring, for 4 to 5 minutes. Stir in 3 cups water, the sweet potato, rice, orzo, salt, pepper, and turmeric or curry and bring to a simmer over medium-high heat. Cover the pan, reduce the heat to low, and cook for 30 to 35 minutes until all of the liquid is absorbed.

Remove from the heat and fluff the grains. Stir in the scallions and let stand for about 10 minutes before serving.

YIELD: 4 SERVINGS

HELPFUL HINT

Orzo, also called rosa marina, is a rice-shaped pasta sold in the Italian section of the grocery store.

Savory Squash Pilaf

Nutrient-rich winter squash and rice team up to form a simple yet flavorful side dish. It is infinitely more interesting than white rice served with a pat of butter.

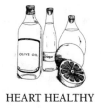

HEART HEALTHY

POWER EATING

1 tablespoon canola oil
1 medium red onion, chopped
2 cloves garlic, minced
3 cups hot water
2 cups diced butternut squash or other winter squash
1½ cups long grain white rice or brown rice
½ teaspoon black pepper
½ teaspoon salt
3 or 4 tablespoons chopped fresh parsley

In a medium saucepan heat the oil over medium heat. Add the onion and garlic and cook, stirring, for 4 minutes. Stir in the water, squash, rice, black pepper, and salt and bring to a simmer. Cover the pan and cook over low heat for 15 to 20 minutes, until all of the liquid is absorbed. (If using brown rice, add ¼ cup more water and cook for 30 to 35 minutes.)

Fluff the rice and stir in the parsley. Let stand (covered) for 10 to 15 minutes before serving.

YIELD: 4 SERVINGS

HELPFUL HINT

Serving this pilaf as a side dish to chicken or fish is a tasty way to increase the overall nutrients of the meal.

Italian-Braised Rapini with Tomatoes

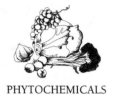

Rapini, also called broccoli rabe, is a leafy green with miniature broccoli florets and a sharp, mustardy flavor. Other greens such as escarole, dandelion greens, or turnip greens can also be braised with garlic and tomatoes.

2　medium bunches rapini (broccoli rabe)
2　tablespoons canola oil
2　or 3 cloves garlic, minced
3　or 4 slices stale dark bread, cubed
2　ripe tomatoes, diced
Salt and black pepper, to taste
2　tablespoons grated Romano cheese (optional)

Remove the fibrous stems of the rapini and discard. Rinse the rapini in a colander and pat dry.

In a large, wide skillet heat the oil over medium heat. Add the garlic and bread and cook, stirring, for 2 to 3 minutes. Stir in the rapini and tomatoes and cook for 5 to 6 minutes more over medium heat, stirring frequently, until the greens are wilted. Transfer to serving plates and season to taste. If desired, sprinkle with grated cheese.

YIELD: 4 SERVINGS

Lemon-Braised Market Greens with Sunflower Seeds

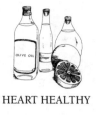

HEART HEALTHY

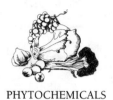

PHYTOCHEMICALS

Farmers' markets around the country offer a bounty of colorful leafy greens. The braising method—cooking the greens with a small amount of liquid (in this case lemon juice)—is one of the easiest ways to prepare leafy greens.

1   large bunch kale, Russian kale, or field spinach
1   tablespoon oil
1   medium onion, finely chopped
2   cloves garlic, minced
Juice of 1 large lemon
$1/2$ teaspoon salt
$1/2$ teaspoon black pepper
1   tablespoon sunflower seeds or sesame seeds

Place the greens in a colander and rinse under cold running water. Remove the stems and coarsely chop the leaves.

In a large skillet heat the oil over medium heat. Add the onion and garlic and cook, stirring, for 2 to 3 minutes. Add the greens, lemon, salt, and pepper and cook for about 4 minutes more over medium-low heat until the greens are wilted.

Transfer the greens to a shallow serving platter. Sprinkle the seeds over the top and serve as a side to grain or pasta dishes.

YIELD: 4 SERVINGS

HELPFUL HINT

Braised greens make a healthful side dish to pilafs, pasta, chicken, and fish entrées.

Tuscan Greens and White Beans

FIBER

Beans and greens form a dynamic combination of healthy nutrients and flavors. A mild green such as escarole is commonly used, but feel free to use your favorite leafy green.

HEART HEALTHY

1 tablespoon olive oil
1 medium yellow onion, chopped
2 or 3 cloves garlic, minced
4 cups coarsely chopped escarole or spinach
3 tablespoons dry wine
1 teaspoon ground sage
$1/2$ teaspoon salt
$1/4$ teaspoon dried red pepper flakes
1 can (15 ounces) white or red kidney beans, drained
$1/4$ cup chopped fresh basil

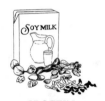

PROTEIN

In a large saucepan heat the oil over medium-high heat. Add the onion and garlic and cook, stirring, for 4 minutes. Add the greens, wine, sage, salt, and red pepper and cook for 3 or 4 more minutes over medium-low heat, stirring frequently, until the greens are wilted. Stir in the beans and basil and cook for 3 minutes more until steaming. Remove from the heat and serve as a hearty side dish.

PHYTOCHEMICALS

YIELD: 4 SERVINGS

Wine-Braised Kale with Wild Mushrooms

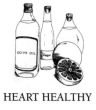

HEART HEALTHY

Verdant kale makes a nutritious companion to earthy mushrooms. Other greens such as Red Russian kale, escarole, or amaranth greens can also be used.

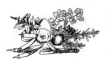

FIRE AND SPICE

1 medium bunch kale (about 1 pound)
1 tablespoon olive oil
3 tablespoons dry white wine
8 ounces button mushrooms, sliced
4 ounces fresh wild mushrooms, sliced (such as crimini, oyster, or shiitake)
1 medium red onion, diced
2 or 3 large cloves garlic, minced
1/2 teaspoon black pepper

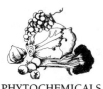

PHYTOCHEMICALS

Remove the fibrous stems from the kale and discard. Rinse the greens in a colander and coarsely chop the leaves.

In a large, wide skillet heat the oil and wine over medium heat. Add the mushrooms, onion, and garlic and cook, stirring, for 6 minutes. Stir in the kale and black pepper and cook for 4 to 5 minutes more over medium heat, stirring frequently, until the greens are wilted.

Transfer the kale and mushrooms to serving plates and serve as a side dish to pasta or pilaf.

YIELD: 4 SERVINGS

Native Squash and Hominy Stew

HEART HEALTHY

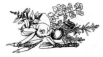

FIRE AND SPICE

Hominy, a kind of dried and puffy corn, makes a chewy addition to this hearty stew of squash, vegetables, and spices.

1 tablespoon canola oil
1 medium yellow onion, diced
1 small zucchini, diced
2 or 3 cloves garlic, minced
1 jalapeño pepper, seeded and minced (optional)
1 can (14 ounces) stewed tomatoes
1 tablespoon dried parsley
2 teaspoons paprika
2 teaspoons dried oregano
$^{1}/_{2}$ teaspoon each black pepper and salt
2 cups peeled, diced butternut squash
1 can (15 ounces) hominy or corn kernels

In a large saucepan heat the oil over medium heat. Add the onion, zucchini, garlic, and jalapeño pepper and cook, stirring, for 4 minutes. Add the tomatoes, parsley, paprika, oregano, pepper, and salt and cook for 3 to 4 minutes more. Add $2^{1}/_{2}$ cups water, the squash, and hominy and cook for 25 to 30 minutes over medium heat, stirring occasionally, until the squash is tender. To thicken the stew, mash the squash against the side of the pan with the back of a spoon. Let stand for 5 to 10 minutes before serving.

Serve in a shallow bowl over brown rice, quinoa, or couscous.

YIELD: 4 TO 6 SERVINGS

HELPFUL HINT

Hominy is available canned or frozen in most well-stocked supermarkets.

Gourmet Squash with Maple Syrup

Gourmet winter squash are easy to prepare, packed with nutrients, and small enough for one or two servings. Some varieties include delicata, sweet dumpling, buttercup, and sugar loaf. This squash dish can be served in place of mashed potatoes.

HEART HEALTHY

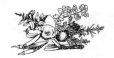

FIRE AND SPICE

3 or 4 delicata squash or other small winter squash
$1/2$ cup soy milk or lowfat milk
1 to 2 tablespoons maple syrup
$1/4$ teaspoon nutmeg
$1/4$ teaspoon white pepper

Preheat the oven to 400 degrees F.

Cut the squash in half lengthwise and scoop out the seeds and stringy fibers. Place the squash cut-side down on a sheet pan filled with about $1/4$-inch water. Bake for 25 to 35 minutes until the flesh is tender (easily pierced with a fork). Remove the squash from the oven, flip over, and let cool for 10 minutes.

When the squash has cooled, scoop out the pulp and transfer to medium mixing bowl. Add the soy milk, maple syrup, nutmeg, and pepper; mash the mixture like potatoes. Serve at once as a healthy side dish.

YIELD: 4 SERVINGS

Pasta with Tomato-Carrot Ragu

Two antioxidant-rich foods—carrots and tomatoes—come together in this robust sauce for pasta.

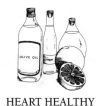

HEART HEALTHY

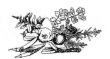

FIRE AND SPICE

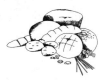

POWER EATING

1   tablespoon canola oil
2   large carrots, chopped
1   medium yellow onion, diced
1   large celery stalk, diced
2   large cloves garlic, minced
1   can (28 ounces) stewed tomatoes
2   tablespoons tomato paste
1   tablespoon dried parsley
2   teaspoons dried oregano
$1/2$ teaspoon black pepper
8   ounces linguini or spaghetti

In a large saucepan heat the oil over medium heat. Add the carrots, onion, celery, and garlic and cook, stirring, until the vegetables are tender, about 6 to 7 minutes. Add the stewed tomatoes, tomato paste, parsley, oregano, and pepper and bring to a simmer. Cook for about 15 minutes over medium-low heat, stirring occasionally. As the sauce cooks, use the edge of a spoon to cut the chunks of tomatoes into smaller pieces.

Meanwhile, in a large saucepan bring 4 quarts of water to a boil over medium-high heat. Place the linguini in the boiling water, stir, and return to a boil. Cook until al dente, 8 to 10 minutes, stirring occasionally. Drain in a colander.

Transfer the linguini to serving plates and ladle the sauce over the top.

YIELD: 4 SERVINGS

Pumpkin-Molasses Muffins

These muffins are a treat you can eat any time of the day.

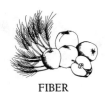
FIBER

¹/₂ cup canola oil
¹/₄ cup applesauce
¹/₂ cup lowfat milk
³/₄ cup brown sugar
1 large egg plus 1 egg white
¹/₄ cup dark molasses
1 can (15 ounces) mashed pumpkin
1 cup diced walnuts
1 cup wheat bran (unprocessed)
1¹/₂ cups unbleached all-purpose flour
1¹/₂ teaspoons baking powder
1 teaspoon ground cinnamon
¹/₂ teaspoon salt

Preheat the oven to 375 degrees F.

Whisk together the oil, applesauce, milk, and sugar in a mixing bowl. Add the eggs and molasses and whisk until the batter is light. Blend in the mashed pumpkin and nuts.

Mix the wheat bran, flour, baking powder, cinnamon, and salt in a separate bowl. Gently fold into pumpkin batter. Spoon the batter into a lightly greased muffin tin and bake for 50 to 60 minutes, until a toothpick inserted in the center comes out clean.

Let cool for about 10 minutes on a rack before serving.

YIELD: 12 MUFFINS

Pillar 2

DISCOVER THE
GOODNESS OF FIBER

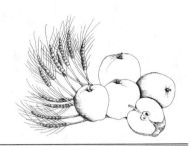

Long on benefits and short on recognition, fiber is finally getting some respect. Although not a glamorous topic or fodder for polite cocktail conversation, fiber plays a major role in the quest for a healthy and fulfilling life. There is a preponderance of evidence documenting the many virtues of a high-fiber, plant-based diet. Fiber-rich foods can promote regularity, relieve constipation, and help to prevent a host of chronic diseases such as colon cancer, heart disease, and obesity. No longer an unsung hero, fiber offers substance over style.

Fiber's health-promoting characteristics are not revolutionary concepts. Most grandmothers knew that apples, cabbage, and beans had something good in them called "roughage" or "bulk," old nicknames for fiber. Not long ago the term "crude fiber" was used to describe the indigestible (and chewy) parts of vegetables, fruits, and other plant foods. Crude fiber evolved into "dietary fiber," and nutritionists now delineate two broad groups of fibers: *water-soluble* and *insoluble*. In addition, numerous kinds of beneficial fiber substances have been identified within each group.

(Pectin, lignin, cellulose, and hemicellulose are some examples.) Our collective understanding of fiber has come a long way from the days of roughage.

Fiber-rich foods are widely available and easy to find in the food supply. From potatoes, tomatoes, apples, and bananas to leafy greens, beans, whole grains, and cereals, there is a cornucopia of good-for-you foods filled with dietary fiber. The supermarket, farmers' market, and country garden are warehouses beckoning with fiber-friendly foods. What's more, you can get all the fiber your body needs from wholesome foods and never, ever have to pop a laxative pill or visit the pharmacy.

While fiber is omnipresent in the plant kingdom, there is absolutely no fiber derived from animal foods. Beef, pork, poultry, fish, eggs, and whole milk contain plenty of cholesterol and saturated fat, but exactly zero fiber. Furthermore, refined foods such as white bread, white rice, french fries, and sugary cereals are stripped of essential fiber during the refining process. It should come as no surprise that the typical American meat-based diet is woefully lacking in disease-preventing fiber.

What exactly is fiber? Why is a high-fiber diet such a great thing? First, about fiber: it refers to the structural substances of plant foods that our bodies cannot digest. Fibrous substances tend to be chewy or crunchy, like the stringy part of celery or the skin of an apple or baked potato. Even though we chew and swallow the fibrous parts of beans, broccoli, cabbage, and so forth, our bodies lack the necessary enzymes to break the fiber down any further. (A cow, with four stomachs, can digest cellulose, but alas, we humans cannot.) Generally speaking, dietary fiber passes through our bodies relatively unchanged.

Since fiber is neither digested nor absorbed, it is technically considered to be a "non-nutrient," a term that is a bit of a misnomer. Although the fibrous parts of plants pass through our bodies undigested, there is a multitude of life-enhancing, disease-preventing attributes linked to a high-fiber diet. In fact, fiber is one of the most important ingredients in the recipe for a healthy life.

- Dietary fiber is found only in plant foods. The goal is to eat a variety of fiber-rich whole foods on a daily basis.
- There is no fiber in meat, chicken, dairy products, or seafood.
- A high-fiber diet may reduce the risk of colon cancer, diverticulosis, and hemorrhoids.
- Soluble fiber may lower the "bad" cholesterol if a low-fat diet is adhered to and thereby reduce the risk of heart disease.
- By providing a slow release of sugar into the bloodstream, fiber helps smooth out blood sugar levels—good news for diabetics and high-performance athletes.
- Fiber is calorie free.
- Cooking has a negligible effect on the amount of fiber contained in food.
- Fiber-rich foods also tend to contain antioxidants, phytonutrients, and energy-giving complex carbohydrates.

THE ALL-STAR VIRTUES OF FIBER

Fiber reduces the body's exposure to harmful food toxins. By adding bulk to our intestinal contents and speeding up the movement of waste through our bodies, fiber accelerates the transit time and facilitates the elimination process. By expediting the elimination cycle, fiber reduces the body's exposure to potential carcinogens and harmful toxins present in some of the foods we eat. The quicker out, the better.

It is well known in the nutrition world that eating a high-fiber diet with plenty of liquids is the best way to prevent and/or treat constipation. Fiber-rich foods increase the bulk and frequency of elimination and effectively reduce the onset of constipation. In addition, fiber-rich foods are a cheaper and healthier alternative to laxatives or fiber supplements.

Fiber helps keep the digestive system "in shape" and thereby helps prevent diverticulosis, a painful condition stemming from weakened and inflamed intestinal walls. It has been estimated that one out of three Americans over the age of 50 suffers from diverticulosis.

A high-fiber diet reduces the risk of colon cancer. There is substantial evidence linking a diet high in insoluble fiber with the reduced risk of colon cancer. Insoluble fiber is believed to inhibit the growth of precancerous polyps. By expediting the elimination of waste, fiber also reduces potential exposure to carcinogens in the foods we eat. Colon cancer is a leading cause of death in Western countries but is relatively rare in countries where high-fiber, plant-based diets are consumed.

Fiber also reduces the risk of heart disease. Studies have shown that a lowfat diet rich in soluble fiber can reduce the level of artery-clogging bad cholesterol (LDL) circulating in the blood. How fiber lowers bad cholesterol is still under investigation, but the end result—reduced levels of cholesterol—is an important step in the effort to curtail the risk of heart disease and stroke.

Since fiber keeps your body feeling "regular" and reduces the occurrence of constipation and hemorrhoids, a high-fiber diet contributes to an overall feeling of well-being. Equanimity prevails when fiber-rich meals are a mainstay, not an exception.

Fiber helps to win the battle of weight control. Fiber-rich foods take longer to chew and digest, thus leaving you with a sated feeling. There is decreased desire to overeat; you feel full for a longer period of time. High-fiber foods also tend to be low in fat and calories. In fact, fiber alone contains zero calories.

Fiber reduces the body's exposure to harmful food toxins, prevents constipation, reduces the occurrence of diverticulosis, reduces the risk of colon cancer and heart disease, contributes to a better quality of life, and helps to win the battle of weight control.

AN IN-DEPTH LOOK AT INSOLUBLE AND SOLUBLE FIBERS

The two main groups of dietary fiber, insoluble and water-soluble, each play important roles in disease prevention. Both types of fiber are found in varied proportions in all kinds of plant foods; certain foods are better sources of one type of fiber than the other. It is important to note that our bodies need an ample amount of both soluble and insoluble fibers, and like antioxidants, the family of fibers works together as a team.

Here is an overview of the two main groups of fibers.

Insoluble Fiber

Insoluble fiber is best described as the coarse, chewy part of plant foods. Examples include the peel of an apple or pear, the skin of a potato, and coarse flakes of unprocessed wheat bran. Previously called roughage or cellulose, insoluble fiber is responsible for relieving constipation, promoting (and improving) regularity, and stimulating the intestinal muscles. Insoluble fiber does not dissolve in water but rather retains and *absorbs water like a sponge* and increases in bulk. Cellulose, lignan, and hemicellulose are some kinds of insoluble fibers.

One of insoluble fiber's greatest attributes is that it shortens the transit time of digested food through the intestines. By easing the movement of waste, insoluble fiber is thought to reduce exposure to potential carcinogens. By limiting the body's exposure to toxins, insoluble fiber may prevent the occurrence of colon cancer. Insoluble fiber also is instrumental in preventing and/or treating diverticulosis, a painful intestinal disorder.

Good sources of insoluble fiber include whole grains, wheat bran, root vegetables with skins, dark leafy greens, bran cereals, unpeeled fruits, nuts, and muffins made with unprocessed bran or wheat germ.

Soluble Fiber

Soluble fiber, also called water-soluble fiber, refers to the indigestible parts of plant foods that dissolve in water. The texture of soluble fibers is sticky and gummy; think of the soft, mushy inside of a cooked kidney bean, prune, or banana. The family of soluble fibers includes pectins, gums, hemicelluloses, and mucilages.

Soluble fiber has an impressive résumé of healthful benefits. Studies have linked soluble fiber with lowering blood cholesterol levels (remember the oat bran craze?). By hindering the production

> **LOOKING FOR FIBER IN ALL THE RIGHT PLACES**
>
> These foods are good sources of dietary fiber:
>
> **The Legume Family:** Black beans, chick-peas, red kidney beans, lentils, pinto beans, split peas, black-eyed peas, and soy beans
>
> **Whole Grain Staples:** Brown rice, quinoa, bulgur, barley, whole wheat couscous, whole wheat pasta, and buckwheat noodles
>
> **Morning Fare:** Bran cereals, bran muffins, oatmeal, and whole grain breads.
>
> **Vegetables and Fruits:** Cruciferous vegetables, winter squash, unpeeled apples, leafy greens, carrots, potatoes, berries, and tropical fruits (kiwi, mango).

Good sources of soluble fiber include apples, bananas, oranges (and other citrus fruits), prunes, carrots, beans, split peas, lentils, oatmeal, oat bran, corn, brown rice, and barley.

of LDL (bad) cholesterol, soluble fiber reduces the risk of heart disease and stroke and fights the buildup of plaque. The theory is that soluble fiber somehow binds or prevents the recycling of cholesterol in the body and thus reduces the overall supply of cholesterol.

In addition, meals high in soluble fiber help the body regulate insulin production and prevent the blood sugar level from darting up rapidly after a meal. This slow, gradual release of sugar into the bloodstream may help diabetics control their blood sugar levels and also contributes to an even flow of energy.

TAPPING INTO THE BENEFITS OF FIBER

How can you benefit from fiber's protective qualities? For starters, eat more fiber-rich foods. Include a variety of legumes, whole grains, wholesome vegetables, fruits (both fresh and dried), and bran cereals in your diet. When shopping for food, take a pass on the refined food products; instead, buy whole wheat bread, brown rice, apples, oranges, and bran muffins. Fill your plate with more

These food sources contain little or no fiber. In addition, the animal foods are high in saturated fat and dietary cholesterol.

Animal Products: Beef, chicken, turkey, pork, seafood, eggs, and processed meat products (cold cuts, bacon, sausages).

Processed Foods: Potato chips, tortilla chips, taco shells, and other snack foods.

Fast Foods: Hamburgers, cheeseburgers, french fries, fried chicken, and fish sticks.

Refined Breads, Cereals, and "Instant" Meals: White bread, instant rice, instant mashed potatoes, and sugary cereals.

vegetables and grains, bean salads and pilafs, and eat less of fiber-deficient meals with meat, chicken, and fish.

It is easy to boost your dietary intake of fiber. After all, fiber is not a scarce commodity in the food chain; it is not some rare and exotic plant substance found only in the Brazilian rain forest. Supermarkets, natural food stores, and backyard gardens are full of fiber-friendly staples.

The edible choices are wide, diverse, and filled with culinary potential. Beans, split peas, and lentils are all well-known powerhouses of fiber. There is an array of fiber-hardy beans including black beans, kidney beans, chick-peas, navy beans, and black-eyed peas. Specialty legumes such as red lentils, appaloosa beans, Jacob's cattle beans, anasazi beans, and adzuki beans are showing up in progressive supermarkets and natural food stores. Other good sources of fiber include grains such as whole wheat, oatmeal, corn, and of course, brown rice and mahogany-hued rices.

AMERICA'S FIBER CRISIS

Despite the vast reservoir of fiber-rich staples available, the diets of most Americans are notoriously lacking in fiber. In fact, it has been estimated that a majority of Americans consume less than *half* of the recommended daily amount of fiber. *Half!* Most people consume only 10–12 grams of fiber a day—a drop in the bucket compared to the 25–35 grams recommended by nutritionists. Clearly, Americans should be eating more fiber-rich foods.

The crux of the problem is that the typical American diet revolves around processed foods. The more processed and refined the food, the lower the fiber content. When wheat flour, rice, and potatoes are refined and polished, valuable fiber is lost in the process. An orange has more fiber than orange juice; brown rice has more fiber than white rice; wheat bread is superior to white bread; and an unpeeled baked potato puts to shame a serving of french fries. For the most part, fiber has been squeezed out of the typical Western diet.

Meanwhile, our fiber-deficient population is besieged with advertisements for constipation aids, laxatives, and digestive aids—a booming industry in this country and a glaring symptom of the low-fiber culture. The evening news is full of commercials for laxatives, hemorrhoids, and fiber supplements. Bouts with irregularity have become an America institution—a phenomenon exacerbated by low-fiber diets.

Why Laxatives and Fiber Pills Miss Their Mark

Americans spend almost a billion dollars a year on constipation aids and laxatives. Digestive aids and fiber supplements address the obvious symptoms of irregularity but do not address the underlying causes—usually a poor diet. Over-the-counter remedies may provide short-term relief but lack the variety of healthy substances found in fiber-rich whole foods. You can't get this vital and complex blend of fibers from a pill or supplement drink.

There are additional health bonuses to eating fiber-rich whole foods. Most foods containing fiber also tend to be low in fat and calories and a good source of complex carbohydrates. Furthermore, when you switch to a high-fiber diet, your body also benefits from an increase in antioxidants and phytonutrients present in many fiber-rich foods.

In the long run, eating a variety of fiber-rich whole foods is the best prescription. A high-fiber diet would alleviate most cases of constipation and irregularity and prevent many life-threatening diseases.

ELEVEN EASY WAYS TO BOOST YOUR FIBER INTAKE

1. Eat the skins and stalks of fruits and vegetables. Don't peel apples, pears, potatoes, and sweet potatoes—there is valuable fiber in the skin. An unpeeled apple has twice as much fiber as a peeled apple. Choose a baked potato over french fries.
2. Choose dark leafy greens over iceberg lettuce. Darker greens have plenty more fiber and nutrients than iceberg lettuce.
3. If you are a recent convert to the high-fiber lifestyle, go slowly at first. Make gradual increases in fiber consumption to give your digestive system (and bacteria and flora) time to adapt. A rapid increase may lead to gastric distress.
4. Choose bran flakes over corn flakes, bran cereal over sugary cereals, and "old-fashioned" oatmeal over instant oatmeal.
5. Include more whole grains in your diet. Brown rice, mahogany rice, and bulgur have appealing textures and flavors. Brown rice only takes 10 to 15 minutes longer to cook than white rice.
6. Eat more beans, even if it means stocking up on canned beans. Add a variety of beans to pasta dishes and sauces (marinara), soups, tossed salads, rice dishes, dips, and casseroles. Choose hummus over sour cream dip, black bean soup over French onion soup, and red beans and rice instead of plain rice.
7. Snack on dried fruits such as apricots, raisins, dates, figs, and prunes. Dried fruits are concentrated sources of fiber.
8. Limit your consumption of fast food meals. Most are notoriously lacking in fiber.

9. When eating high-fiber foods, drink plenty of water. Fluids ease the absorption of fiber.
10. Choose dark breads over white bread. Whole wheat, pumpernickel, and multigrain breads contain more fiber than refined breads.
11. Start your day with a high-fiber breakfast cereal. If your favorite cereal is low in fiber, mix in a high-fiber bran cereal—there are plenty of brands to choose from.

A diversified, plant-based diet is the best path to creating long-term health and well-being. Increasing the amount of fiber in your diet is one of most important dietary changes you can make in your life.

GET JUMP-STARTED WITH FIBER

If you are not currently on a high-fiber diet but would like to increase your fiber intake—which is a good idea—it is best to do it *gradually*. Eat a variety of fiber-rich foods and spread your consumption over the course of the day. Too much fiber eaten too quickly may cause a bloated sensation and gastric distress. (Your intestines will need time to adjust.) Also, drink plenty of water to help your body accommodate the increase in fiber-rich foods (remember, insoluble fiber absorbs water like a sponge).

There is still much to be learned about fiber's role in preventing disease and promoting health. Although the evidence is accumulating, the scientific community is not one hundred percent in agreement that fiber acts alone in preventing disease. Some believe that fiber is a marker for other substances present in fiber-rich whole foods. It could be that fiber works with other plant substances yet to be identified. All in all, focusing on fiber is an important element in the quest for a healthy life.

FIBER IN THE KITCHEN

Legumes

Legumes include the diverse family of dried beans, split peas, and lentils. Legumes are good sources dietary fiber, protein, iron, calcium, and complex carbohydrates. In addition, legumes are naturally low in fat, calories, and sodium. Versatile and economical, legumes add substance, texture, and flavor to almost any meal, from hearty soups, salads, and grain dishes to breakfast fare and vegetable dips. Legumes also take a long time to digest and provide a full, satisfied feeling after a meal.

Here are a few tips for cooking with legumes.

Preparation: Before cooking, dried beans must be sorted for pebbles and soaked in plenty of water for at least 4 hours (preferably overnight). After soaking, drain the beans and cook them in plenty of fresh water. Most beans take an hour or more to become tender; lentils take about 45 minutes.

Cooking Tips: To produce tender and plump beans, avoid adding salt or acidic ingredients (such as tomatoes or vinegar) to the bean pot during the cooking process (salt and acid inhibit water absorption). Stir the beans occasionally, and cook over medium-low heat.

Canned Beans: When you don't have time to cook dried beans from scratch, include canned beans in your culinary repertoire. Canned beans are convenient, widely available, and easy to store. Look for canned beans with reduced sodium content and processed without sugar. About 1½ cups of cooked beans can replace one 15-ounce can of beans in most recipes throughout this book.

A Cook's Guide to Legumes

Legumes come in multiple shapes, sizes, and colors. Here is a description of some popular legumes that can be found in the healthful pantry. Most supermarkets and natural food stores carry a wide selection of familiar and exotic legumes.

Adzuki Beans, also called aduki beans, are small, burgundy red beans with a nutty, slightly sweet flavor. Popular in Asian cuisine, adzuki beans are often combined with rice for a dish called "red rice." Adzuki beans are also cooked, mashed, and sweetened and used as a filling for Asian pastries, breads, and turnovers.

Anasazi Beans are ancient heirloom beans grown in Colorado and the American Southwest. Anasazi beans have a slight kidney shape and reddish purple skin with creamy mottled streaks. The beans can be added to chili, soups, and hearty stews.

Black Beans are oval, pea-shaped beans with an earthy, woodsy flavor. Popular in Latin American, Caribbean, and Mexican cooking, black beans inspire hearty soups, salads, dips, chilies, and rice dishes. Brazilian feijoada, Cuban beans and rice, and Mexican black bean soup (*sopa feijoa negro*) are some classic black bean dishes.

Black-Eyed Peas are round, creamy white beans with a distinctive dark "eye" on their ridges. They have an earthy, mealy flavor and firm texture. Black-eyed peas are prevalent in the American South, Africa, the Caribbean, and the Middle East. The Southern dish "Hoppin' John" is made with black-eyed peas.

Chick-Peas, also called garbanzo beans or *ceci* beans, are shaped like tiny tan-colored acorns. Popular in Mediterranean, Indian, Caribbean, and Middle Eastern cooking, chick-peas have a chewy texture and a nutty nuance. The versatile beans are used in hummus, pasta dishes, vegetable soups, pilafs, and multi-bean salads.

Cranberry Beans, also called Roman beans, are oval beans with a speckled, beige-and-cranberry skin. Similar to pinto beans in flavor, cranberry beans are common in Italian, Native American, and South American stews and soups.

Lentils come in brown, green, red, orange, black, and yellow colors. The elliptical, disc-shaped lentils cook faster than most legumes and are also easy to digest. Lentils are a mainstay in Indian, Middle Eastern, North African, and European cooking. Lentils are commonly used in Indian dal, vegetable curries, hearty soups, and grain salads.

Pigeon Peas, also called gungo peas, are small, pea-shaped, tannish yellow beans with a tiny eye and faint freckle marks. The pea-shaped beans are a favored legume in Caribbean soups, stews, and grain dishes such as peas-and-rice.

Pinto Beans are mottled, pinkish brown beans with a mealy bean flavor. When cooked, the pinto markings (named after the horse) fade to pink. Pintos are a staple of Mexican, Tex-Mex, Southwestern, and Native American fare (refried beans are made with pinto beans).

Red Kidney Beans are kidney-shaped beans with a rich, meaty flavor and chewy texture. Common varieties include dark red, light red, and white beans. Kidney beans are used in Latin American, Caribbean, and Creole/Cajun cooking and inspire robust chilies, soups, bean-and-rice salads, three-bean salads, vegetable stews, and countless varieties of pilafs.

Soybeans, also called soya beans, are about the size of a large pea. Tannish yellow soybeans are available in America, but Asian varieties include black, green, brown, and red versions. Soybeans are often processed into a variety of soy foods such as soy sauce, tamari, miso, soy milk, soy flour, tofu, tempeh, fermented bean pastes, and soybean oil. Soybeans require a long cooking time—several hours, in fact.

Split Peas are whole green or yellow peas that have been split in half. Well-cooked split peas develop a porridgelike consistency and a wholesome grassy flavor. Split peas are prevalent in Mediterranean, European, Indian, and traditional American meals and are famous for inspiring myriad versions of soothing split pea soup.

White Beans refers to a collection of legumes that includes Great Northern beans, white kidney beans (cannelini beans), and small, oval, navy beans. White beans are prevalent in European cuisines and are used in casseroles, soups, and stews. Boston baked beans and senate bean soup are both prepared with white beans.

TEN STEPS IN THE "BEAN ROUTINE"	1. Toss chick-peas into a leafy green salad.

TEN STEPS IN
THE "BEAN
ROUTINE"

1. Toss chick-peas into a leafy green salad.
2. Add red kidney beans to red sauces for pasta.
3. Stir black beans or red beans into salsa.
4. Add red or white kidney beans to tomato-based soups (such as minestrone).
5. For pilafs, add chick-peas, black-eyed peas, or black beans to the rice while it cooks.
6. For a quick bean salad, combine two or three kinds of beans together with vinaigrette dressing, garlic, and fresh herbs. Add artichokes, corn, or tomatoes.
7. For variety, try black beans or white beans in chili and leave out the meat.
8. Add sturdy chick-peas to long-cooking stews and curries.
9. Add chick-peas and red beans to pasta salads and potato salads
10. Add black beans and black-eyed peas to rice salads and grain salads.

Whole Grains

Whole grains are good sources of fiber, antioxidants, and complex carbohydrates. When grains are combined with legumes a complete protein is formed. Unlike "refined" grain products such as white rice and white flour, minimally processed whole grains contain much of their natural fiber.

The problem with white rice and refined grains is that the nutrient-dense bran layer has been removed during the milling process. However, white rice does not have to be completely abandoned; the goal is to increase the meal's fiber content by adding other healthful staples such as cooked beans, lentils, cracked wheat, or seasonal vegetables to the dish.

A Cook's Guide to High-Fiber Grains

There are a number of delicious grains, each with a unique flavor and consistency, commonly available in well-stocked supermarkets.

Brown Rice is a beige-colored whole grain rice with its outer bran layer intact. Brown rice has a nutty flavor, a chewy texture, and twice the fiber of polished white rice. Brown rice takes about 35 to 40 minutes to cook and requires slightly more liquid than white rice. Brown rice can replace white rice in many recipes.

Bulgur refers to whole wheat berries that have been precooked, dried, and cracked. To cook bulgur, steep the tiny grains in hot water for about fifteen minutes (like couscous). Bulgur can be used in pilafs, salads, cold soups, and tabbouleh.

Cracked Wheat refers to processed whole wheat kernels that are similar to bulgur. However, unlike bulgur, cracked wheat has not been precooked. For the most part, cracked wheat and bulgur are interchangeable.

Oat Bran inspired a diet craze in the 1980s, when soluble fiber was associated with reduced levels of cholesterol. An explosion of oat bran muffins, breads, cookies, cereals, snacks—even oat bran beer—hit the market. The frenzy subsided when it was learned that *reducing the saturated fat and cholesterol* in one's diet remained the best way to reduce the risk of heart attack—not eating a bowl of oat bran for every meal. However, oat bran still has a place in the healthful diet. The bran can be used like wheat bran in most recipes.

Oatmeal makes an excellent hot breakfast dish. Don't ruin a bowl of hot oatmeal by adding butter or cream to the dish; maple syrup, fresh fruit, and puréed fruit are healthful toppings. In addition, sprinkle oatmeal flakes over muffins, breads, or cold cereals. Oatmeal is sold as "rolled" and "quick cooking," which are partially cooked.

Whole Wheat Couscous is made from durum wheat, the grain used to make spaghetti. Couscous cooks up in about ten minutes and can be tossed with other grains, beans, and sautéed vegetables. Wheat couscous is interchangeable with refined couscous.

Wild Rice is not really a rice, but a dark, slender seed of a native North American aquatic grass. The grain has a firm, chewy texture and a grassy flavor. Wild rice is harvested in the northern lakes of Minnesota and Canada. Due to its strong flavor (and high price), wild rice is ideally blended with other rices and grains. It cooks in about 45 to 50 minutes.

Wheat

Wheat is one of the most widely cultivated crops in the world. Wheat products are found in everything from breads and cereals to pastas, salads, and baked goods. The versatile cereal grain is processed and sold as wheat berries, bran and bran flakes, wheat germ, cracked wheat, bulgur, farina, whole wheat flour, and bread.

It is the bran layer—the outermost layer of the wheat grain— that supplies a mother lode of nutrients and dietary fiber. Bran is a solid source of insoluble fiber as well as protein, iron, and niacin. Wheat bran is readily available in breakfast cereals, bran muffins, and baked goods that include whole wheat flour. (To produce white flour, the bran layer is removed during the refining process. As a result, white bread and other products made exclusively with white flour are low in fiber.)

I am continually amazed by the number of people who buy white bread. White bread is mushy and flimsy and exhibits a bleached taste. Most brands of whole wheat bread have more fiber and superior flavor and texture. However, when buying commercial wheat breads, *read the label.* Some brands labeled "wheat bread" are really white bread that has been dyed with caramel coloring. *Whole wheat flour* should be the first ingredient listed.

A Cook's Guide to Wheat Products
Here is a description of the many wheat and grain products available in well-stocked grocery stores and natural food stores.

Bran Cereal usually refers to wheat flakes or crumbled wheat "strands." Bran cereals are good sources of fiber and other nutrients. Choose bran cereals that list bran as the number-one ingredient—and avoid brands that list a sweetener (such as corn syrup, sugar, or fructose) as a main ingredient. Eating a bowl of bran cereal with fruit is an excellent way to start the day.

Wheat Berries are whole kernels of wheat. Like beans, wheat berries should be soaked for several hours prior to cooking. They take two to three hours to cook and will absorb a lot of water, so be sure to include enough.

Wheat Bran refers to the outer layer of the wheat kernel. Bran adds fiber to breads, cereals, muffins, and other baked goods. Also called bran or unprocessed bran, wheat bran is a great source of fiber, protein, iron, and B vitamins. Although wheat bran is the most available bran product, other forms include rice bran, oat bran, and corn bran.

Wheat Germ is the "germ" of the wheat seed. Wheat germ has a strong, wheaty flavor. It can be blended (in moderate amounts) into muffins, breads, pancakes, fruit shakes, and baked goods. Wheat germ can also be sprinkled over cold or hot cereals. It is a good source of fiber, protein, vitamin E, iron, and B vitamins.

Whole Wheat Flour is a brownish and heavy flour that is ideally blended with unbleached white flour in baking recipes. When used by itself, whole wheat flour yields a dense, dry baked product. Combining whole wheat flour with white flour yields a fluffier and more leavened product. That is one way to strike a balance between lofty health goals and amiable tastes and textures.

Whole Wheat Pasta cooks up just like refined pasta and contains twice the fiber. Whole wheat pasta offers a nice change of pace from refined pasta and cooks in about half the time.

SIGNATURE RECIPES FOR THE FIBER-RICH, HEALTHY DIET

Black Bean Sofrito

Piquant Black Bean Dip

Sweet Pepper Hummus

White Bean and Corn Chili

Brown Rice and Two-Bean Chili

Super Bowl of Red

Country Black Bean Soup

Southwestern Pasta Fazool

Tangy Black-Eyed Pea and Bulgur Salad

Garden Three-Bean Salad

Pasta and Artichoke Salad with Chick-Peas

White Beans and Greens

Red Lentil–Potato Dal

Green and Red Bean Tureen

Black-Eyed Pea, Greens, and Bulgur Pilaf

Curried Chick-Peas with Potatoes

Dill Potatoes and Carrots with Chick-Peas

Veggie Bran Raisin Muffins

Banana-Blueberry Bran Bread

Pumpkin Fruit Pancakes with Oat Bran

Apple Berry Cake

Additional health benefits are noted with each recipe.

Black Bean Sofrito

Sofrito is a versatile Hispanic condiment of sautéed vegetables and herbs. As a topping, sofrito can take the place of sour cream or butter in rice, pilaf, soup, baked potatoes, and other mild dishes in need of a pick-me-up.

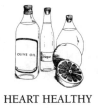

HEART HEALTHY

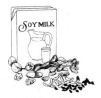

PROTEIN

1 tablespoon canola oil
1 medium yellow onion, diced
1 green or red bell pepper, seeded and diced
2 cloves garlic, minced
1 can (15 ounces) black beans, drained
1 can (14 ounces) stewed tomatoes
1 teaspoon dried oregano
1/2 teaspoon ground cumin
1/2 teaspoon black pepper
1/2 teaspoon salt
2 to 3 tablespoons chopped fresh cilantro

In a medium saucepan heat the oil over medium-high heat. Add the onion, bell pepper, and garlic and cook, stirring, for 5 to 6 minutes. Add the beans, tomatoes, oregano, cumin, pepper, and salt and cook for 7 to 10 minutes more over low heat, stirring frequently. Stir in the cilantro and remove from the heat.

Spoon the sofrito over rice, potatoes, squash, or other grain dishes.

YIELD: 4 TO 6 SERVINGS

Piquant Black Bean Dip

HEART HEALTHY

PROTEIN

This spicy, fiber-rich dip is a much better choice to serve than any hackneyed sour cream concoction made with a sodium-laden French onion soup mix.

1 tablespoon canola oil
1 small yellow onion, diced
1 cubanelle pepper or bell pepper, seeded and diced
1 tomato, diced
2 cloves garlic, minced
1 to 2 jalapeño peppers, seeded and minced
2 cans (15 ounces each) black beans, drained
2 large scallions, chopped
1 1/2 teaspoons dried oregano
1 teaspoon ground cumin
1/2 teaspoon black pepper
1/2 teaspoon salt
1 to 2 teaspoons bottled hot sauce (to taste)

In a medium saucepan heat the oil over medium heat. Add the onion, bell pepper, tomato, garlic, and jalapeños and cook, stirring, for 5 minutes. Add the beans, scallions, oregano, cumin, pepper, and salt and cook for 7 to 10 minutes more over low heat, stirring occasionally.

Let the mixture cool slightly. Transfer to a food processor fitted with a steel blade or to a blender and process until smooth, about 5 to 10 seconds. Pour the puréed beans into a serving bowl, mix in hot sauce, and serve with warm flour tortillas or pita bread. (If serving later, the dip can be refrigerated for up to three days. Reheat before serving.)

YIELD: ABOUT 4 CUPS

Sweet Pepper Hummus

Sweet red peppers give this classic dip of pureed chick-peas an uplifting flavor and inviting hue.

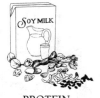

PROTEIN

^{1}/4 cup diced roasted sweet peppers (from a jar)
1 can (15 ounces) chick-peas, drained
^{1}/2 cup plain lowfat yogurt
^{1}/4 cup tahini (sesame seed paste)
Juice of 1 lemon
2 cloves garlic, minced
^{1}/2 teaspoon ground cumin
^{1}/2 teaspoon black pepper
^{1}/4 teaspoon salt
3 or 4 tablespoons chopped fresh parsley

Put all of the ingredients except the parsley in a food processor fitted with a steel blade or in a blender and process for 10 to 15 seconds, until smooth. Transfer to a serving bowl and garnish with the parsley.

Serve with warm pita bread and raw vegetables such as carrots, celery, sweet peppers, and broccoli. The hummus also makes a tasty sandwich spread.

YIELD: ABOUT 2 CUPS

White Bean and Corn Chili

This inventive meatless chili abounds with fiber, protein, and healthful flavors.

ANTIOXIDANTS

HEART HEALTHY

PROTEIN

1 tablespoon canola oil
2 tomatoes, diced
1 large yellow onion, diced
1 yellow or red bell pepper, seeded and diced
2 cups diced eggplant
2 large cloves garlic, minced
1½ cups corn kernels, fresh or frozen
1 can (15 ounces) white kidney beans, drained
1 can (15 ounces) crushed tomatoes
2 teaspoons dried oregano
2 teaspoons chili powder
1½ teaspoons ground cumin
½ teaspoon salt
½ teaspoon black pepper

In a large saucepan heat the oil over medium heat. Add the diced tomatoes, onion, bell pepper, eggplant, and garlic and cook over medium heat for 8 to 10 minutes, stirring occasionally. Stir in the corn, beans, crushed tomatoes, oregano, chili powder, cumin, salt, and pepper and bring to a simmer. Cook (uncovered) for about 20 minutes over low heat, stirring occasionally.

Remove the chili from the heat and let stand for 5 minutes before serving. Ladle into bowls and serve with cornbread.

YIELD: 6 SERVINGS

Brown Rice and Two-Bean Chili

You won't miss the meat in this spicy chili of whole grain rice, beans, and vegetables.

ANTIOXIDANTS

2 teaspoons canola oil
1 medium yellow onion, diced
1 green bell pepper, seeded and diced
2 stalks celery, diced
4 cloves garlic, minced
1 can (28 ounces) stewed tomatoes, undrained
1 can (15 ounces) red kidney beans, drained
1 can (15 ounces) pinto beans, drained
1½ cups corn kernels, frozen or canned
1 cup uncooked brown rice
2 tablespoons chili powder
1 tablespoon dried oregano
1½ teaspoons ground cumin
½ teaspoon each black pepper and salt

HEART HEALTHY

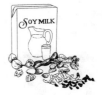

PROTEIN

In a large saucepan heat the oil over medium-high heat. Add the onion, bell pepper, celery, and garlic and cook, stirring, for 7 minutes. Stir in the stewed tomatoes, beans, corn, 2 cups water, rice, chili powder, oregano, cumin, pepper, and salt and bring to a simmer. Cover and cook over medium-low heat for 35 to 40 minutes until the rice is tender, stirring occasionally. Remove the chili from the heat and let stand for 10 minutes before serving.

Ladle into bowls and serve with fresh bread.

POWER EATING

YIELD: 6 SERVINGS

HELPFUL HINT

Offer lowfat yogurt as a topping.

Super Bowl of Red

ANTIOXIDANTS

This meatless "party" chili is unpretentious and exuberantly spiced. Serve it with a selection of toppings such as chopped scallions, shredded cheese, chopped red onions, and/or lowfat yogurt.

HEART HEALTHY

PROTEIN

1 tablespoon canola oil
1 large yellow onion, diced
2 green or red bell peppers, seeded and diced
2 stalks celery, diced
4 cloves garlic, minced
1 can (28 ounces) crushed tomatoes
1 can (15 ounces) red kidney beans, drained
1 can (14 ounces) stewed tomatoes
1 tablespoon chili powder
1 tablespoon dried oregano
2 teaspoons ground cumin
1 teaspoon paprika
1 teaspoon salt
1 to 2 teaspoons Tabasco or other bottled hot sauce
1/2 teaspoon black pepper

In a large saucepan heat the oil over medium-high heat. Add the onion, bell peppers, celery, and garlic and sauté, stirring, for 6 to 8 minutes, until the vegetables are tender. Stir in the crushed tomatoes, beans, stewed tomatoes, chili powder, oregano, cumin, paprika, salt, hot sauce, and pepper and bring to a simmer. Cook for 25 to 30 minutes (uncovered) over low heat, stirring occasionally. Remove from the heat and let stand for 5 to 10 minutes before serving.

Ladle the chili into bowls and serve with cornbread or whole wheat bread.

YIELD: 4 TO 6 SERVINGS

HELPFUL HINT

If you would like to add meat to this chili, add about $1/2$ pound of diced lean sirloin after the vegetables have been sautéing for three minutes. Do *not* add fatty ground beef or chuck.

Country Black Bean Soup

ANTIOXIDANTS

This wholesome black bean soup resonates with nourishing flavors and inviting textures.

1 1/2 cups dried black beans, soaked overnight and drained
1 tablespoon canola oil
1 large yellow onion, diced
1 red bell pepper, seeded and diced
1 large stalk celery, chopped
3 to 4 cloves garlic, minced
1 jalapeño pepper, seeded and minced
2 medium carrots or 1 sweet potato, diced
1 tablespoon dried oregano
1 1/2 teaspoons cumin
1 teaspoon coriander
1 teaspoon dried thyme
1/2 teaspoon black pepper
1/2 cup canned crushed tomatoes
1/2 teaspoon salt
2 tablespoons chopped fresh cilantro

HEART HEALTHY

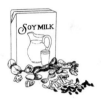

PROTEIN

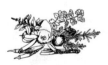

FIRE AND SPICE

In a medium saucepan combine the beans and 6 cups water and bring to a simmer. Cook for 1 to 1 1/2 hours over medium-low heat until the beans are tender. Drain the beans, reserving 4 cups of the cooking liquid.

In a large saucepan heat the oil over medium-high heat. Add the onion, bell pepper, celery, garlic, and jalapeño and cook, stirring, for 5 minutes. Add the beans, cooking liquid, carrots, oregano, cumin, coriander, thyme, and pepper. Bring to a simmer and cook for about 20 minutes over medium-low heat, stirring occasionally.

Stir in the crushed tomatoes, salt, and cilantro. Cook for 10 to 15 minutes more, stirring occasionally. Remove from the heat and let stand for 10 minutes. (If you prefer a thick soup, purée half of the soup in a food processor fitted with a steel blade and return to the pan.)

Ladle the soup into bowls. If desired, serve with flour tortillas.

YIELD: 6 TO 8 SERVINGS

HELPFUL HINT

Soak the beans in plenty of water before cooking. After draining, cook the beans in fresh water.

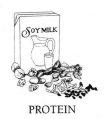

PROTEIN

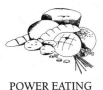

POWER EATING

Southwestern Pasta Fazool

This twist on the classic Italian bean soup exudes adventurous flavors.

1 tablespoon canola oil
1 medium yellow onion, diced
1 red or green bell pepper, seeded and diced
4 cloves garlic, minced
1 or 2 jalapeño peppers, seeded and minced
6 cups vegetable broth
$1/2$ cup canned tomato paste
2 teaspoons dried oregano
$1^1/2$ teaspoons ground cumin
$1/2$ teaspoon black pepper
$1/2$ teaspoon salt
1 cup elbow macaroni
1 can (11 ounces) corn kernels, drained
1 cup cooked black beans or red kidney beans
2 tablespoons chopped fresh cilantro

In a large saucepan heat the oil over medium-high heat. Add the onion, bell pepper, garlic, and jalapeño and cook, stirring, for 6 minutes. Add the vegetable broth, tomato paste, oregano, cumin, pepper, and salt and bring to a simmer over medium heat, stirring occasionally. Stir in the macaroni, corn, beans, and cilantro and return to a simmer. Cook for 5 to 7 minutes over medium-high heat, stirring occasionally, until the pasta is al dente.

Remove from the heat and let stand for 5 to 10 minutes before serving. Ladle the soup into shallow bowls and serve with warmed flour tortillas.

YIELD: 6 SERVINGS

Tangy Black-Eyed Pea and Bulgur Salad

This grain and bean salad can be served as a stuffing for pita bread or as a refreshing side dish for dinner.

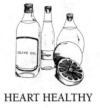

HEART HEALTHY

1 cup bulgur
1 cup boiling water
1 can (15 ounces) black-eyed peas, drained
1 large tomato, diced
1 medium cucumber, chopped (peeled if waxed)
2 or 3 large scallions, chopped
2 cloves garlic, minced
2 tablespoons olive oil
Juice of 1 to 2 lemons
1/4 cup chopped parsley
1/2 teaspoon black pepper
1/2 teaspoon salt

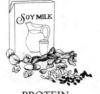

PROTEIN

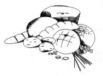

POWER EATING

Combine the bulgur and water in a medium mixing bowl and let soak for 15 to 20 minutes until the bulgur absorbs all of the water.

Meanwhile, in another mixing bowl combine the remaining ingredients and toss together. Blend the bulgur into the black-eyed pea mixture. Chill the salad for at least 1 hour before serving.

Serve the salad as a stuffing for pita bread or on a serving plate lined with green leaf lettuce.

YIELD: 4 SERVINGS

HELPFUL HINT

For an herbal nuance, add 2 or 3 tablespoons of chopped fresh mint.

Garden Three-Bean Salad

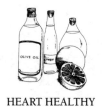

HEART HEALTHY

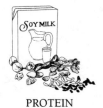

PROTEIN

The classic three-bean salad is reinvigorated with fresh vegetables, garden herbs, and a light vinaigrette dressing.

1 can (15 ounces) chick-peas, drained
1 can (15 ounces) red kidney beans, drained
1 can (15 ounces) black beans or black-eyed peas, drained
1 red bell pepper, seeded and diced
1 large cucumber, diced (peeled if waxed)
4 to 6 scallions, chopped
2 tomatoes, diced
4 cloves garlic, minced
3 tablespoons olive oil
3 tablespoons balsamic vinegar
1/4 cup chopped fresh parsley
2 teaspoons dried oregano
1 teaspoon black pepper
1/2 teaspoon salt

In a large mixing bowl combine all of the ingredients and blend thoroughly. Chill for at least 1 hour before serving.

Serve in a large bowl with leaf lettuce arranged around the rim.

YIELD: 4 TO 6 SERVINGS

HELPFUL HINT

Add a few tablespoons of chopped summer herbs such as basil, arugula, or chives.

Pasta and Artichoke Salad with Chick-Peas

PROTEIN

Artichokes lend a regal presence to this summery pasta and bean salad.

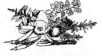

FIRE AND SPICE

- 8 ounces penne or ziti pasta
- 3 tablespoons canola oil
- 3 tablespoons red wine vinegar or balsamic vinegar
- 1 tablespoon Dijon-style mustard
- 1/4 cup chopped fresh parsley
- 2 large cloves garlic, minced
- 2 teaspoons dried oregano
- 1/2 teaspoon black pepper
- 2 ripe tomatoes, diced
- 4 scallions, chopped
- 1 can (15 ounces) chick-peas, drained
- 1 can (14 ounces) artichoke hearts, drained and coarsely chopped

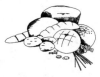

POWER EATING

In a large saucepan bring 2 1/2 quarts of water to a boil over medium-high heat. Place the pasta in the boiling water, stir, and return to a boil. Cook until al dente, about 9 to 11 minutes. Drain in a colander and cool under cold running water.

Meanwhile, in a large mixing bowl whisk together the oil, vinegar, mustard, parsley, garlic, oregano, and pepper. Add the pasta, tomatoes, scallions, chick-peas, and artichokes and blend together. Refrigerate the salad for about 1 hour before serving.

YIELD: 4 SERVINGS

HELPFUL HINT

Toss in a green vegetable such as steamed asparagus, broccoli, or green beans.

White Beans and Greens

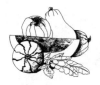

ANTIOXIDANTS

HEART HEALTHY

PROTEIN

PHYTOCHEMICALS

Braised leafy greens make a flavorful companion to hearty white beans. A dash of lemon perks up the dish at the last minute.

2 teaspoons canola oil
1 small yellow onion, finely chopped
2 cloves garlic, minced
2 cups coarsely chopped Russian kale or green kale
2 cups coarsely chopped spinach
1/2 teaspoon black pepper
1/2 teaspoon salt
1 can (15 ounces) white kidney beans, drained
1 lemon, quartered

In a large skillet or wok heat the oil over medium heat. Add the onion and garlic and cook, stirring, for 3 minutes. Add the greens, pepper, and salt and cook, stirring, for 3 to 4 minutes more until the greens are wilted. Blend in the beans and cook for 4 minutes more until the beans are steaming. Squeeze the lemon over the greens and beans and remove from the heat.

Serve as a side dish with grains or pasta.

YIELD: 4 SERVINGS

Red Lentil–Potato Dal

Dal is a comforting Indian dish radiating with warm curry flavors. Cook the lentils and potatoes until they reach a smooth, puréed consistency.

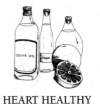

HEART HEALTHY

2 teaspoons canola oil
1 large yellow onion, chopped
3 or 4 cloves garlic, minced
1 large tomato, diced
1¹/2 teaspoons curry powder
¹/2 teaspoon ground cumin
¹/2 teaspoon black pepper
¹/4 teaspoon turmeric
1 cup red lentils, rinsed
2 cups peeled, diced white potatoes or sweet potatoes
¹/2 teaspoon salt

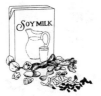

PROTEIN

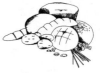

POWER EATING

In a medium saucepan heat the oil over medium heat. Add the onion and garlic and cook, stirring, for about 5 minutes. Stir in the tomato, curry powder, cumin, pepper, and turmeric and cook for 1 minute more. Stir in the lentils and 4 cups water and cook over medium-low heat for 15 minutes, stirring occasionally. Stir in the potatoes and cook for about 30 minutes more, stirring occasionally, until the lentils and potatoes are tender. Stir in the salt and let stand for about 10 minutes.

Transfer the dal to a large serving bowl. Serve with warm Indian flat bread, pita bread, or flour tortillas. Plain yogurt makes a cooling condiment.

YIELD: 4 TO 6 SERVINGS

HELPFUL HINT

For a touch of heat, add 1 hot chili pepper (seeded and minced) while sautéing the onion and garlic.

Green and Red Bean Tureen

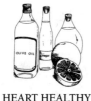

HEART HEALTHY

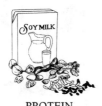

PROTEIN

This healthy Tex-Mex creation beckons with nutritious vegetables.

2 teaspoons canola oil
1 medium yellow onion, diced
1 green bell pepper, seeded and diced
2 stalks celery, diced
3 or 4 cloves garlic, minced
1 can (28 ounces) plum tomatoes
1 can (15 ounces) red kidney beans, drained
1 can (11 ounces) corn kernels, drained
1/3 pound green beans, trimmed and cut into 1-inch pieces
1 tablespoon chili powder
2 teaspoons dried oregano
1/4 teaspoon cayenne pepper
1/2 teaspoon salt

In a large saucepan heat the oil over medium-high heat. Add the onion, bell pepper, celery, and garlic and cook, stirring, for 7 minutes. Stir in the plum tomatoes, red beans, corn, green beans, chili powder, oregano, cayenne, and salt and bring to a simmer. Cook over medium-low heat for 15 minutes, stirring occasionally. (Cut the plum tomatoes into small pieces as you stir.) Let stand for about 5 minutes before serving.

Ladle into bowls and serve with brown rice.

YIELD: 6 SERVINGS

HELPFUL HINT

To perk up the heat, drizzle one or two teaspoons of bottled hot sauce into the pot before serving.

Black-Eyed Pea, Greens, and Bulgur Pilaf

This flavorful pilaf is loaded with fiber, protein, calcium, iron, and phytonutrients.

HEART HEALTHY

2   teaspoons canola oil
1   medium yellow onion, diced
2   cloves garlic, minced
4   cups chopped fresh spinach or green chard
1   can (15 ounces) black-eyed peas, drained
$1/2$ teaspoon salt
$1/2$ teaspoon black pepper
1   cup bulgur (coarse)
$1/4$ cup chopped fresh parsley
1   lemon, cut into wedges

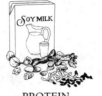

PROTEIN

In a saucepan heat the oil over medium-high heat. Add the onion and garlic and cook, stirring, for about 4 minutes. Add $2^{1}/_2$ cups water, the spinach or chard, black-eyed peas, salt, and pepper and bring to a simmer. Cook for about 4 minutes. Stir in the bulgur and parsley and cover the pan. Let stand for 12 to 15 minutes until all of the liquid is absorbed.

Fluff the grains and squeeze the lemon over the top. Serve as a hearty side dish.

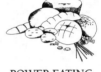

POWER EATING

YIELD: 4 SERVINGS

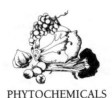

PHYTOCHEMICALS

Curried Chick-Peas with Potatoes

HEART HEALTHY

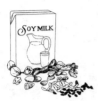

PROTEIN

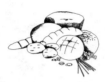

POWER EATING

This satisfying side dish of chick-peas and potatoes exudes aromatic flavors of curry.

1 tablespoon canola oil
1 medium yellow onion, diced
1 large ripe tomato, diced
2 cloves garlic, minced
1 jalapeño or other chili pepper, seeded and minced
1 tablespoon dried parsley
2 to 3 teaspoons curry powder (preferably West Indian)
1 1/2 teaspoons ground cumin
3/4 teaspoon salt
1/2 teaspoon black pepper
2 cups diced white potatoes
1 can (15 ounces) chick-peas, drained

In a large saucepan heat the oil over medium-high heat. Add the onion, tomato, garlic, and jalapeño and cook, stirring, for 5 minutes. Stir in the parsley, curry, cumin, salt, and pepper, reduce the heat to low, and sauté for 1 minute more. Add the potatoes and 2 cups water and cook for 15 minutes over medium heat, stirring occasionally. Stir in the chick-peas and cook for 10 to 15 minutes more until the potatoes are tender. To thicken, mash some of the potatoes against the side of the pan with the back of a large spoon.

Serve the curry vegetables over a pile of rice or other grains.

YIELD: 4 SERVINGS

HELPFUL HINT

To make this a traditional curry dish, add 1/2 pound boneless, diced chicken along with the seasonings.

Dill Potatoes and Carrots with Chick-Peas

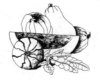

This herb-scented dish of mashed potatoes has a little of everything: fiber, beta-carotene, complex carbohydrates, and soy protein.

4 cups diced white potatoes (preferably unpeeled)
2 large carrots, diced
1 can (15 ounces) chick-peas, drained
$1/2$ cup soy milk or lowfat dairy milk
2 tablespoons chopped fresh parsley
2 cloves garlic, minced
2 large whole scallions, chopped
2 teaspoons dill weed
$1/2$ teaspoon white pepper
$1/4$ teaspoon salt

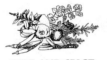

In a medium saucepan bring $2^{1/2}$ quarts of water to a boil. Place the potatoes and carrots in the boiling water and cook for 18 to 20 minutes until the vegetables are easily pierced with a fork. Drain in a colander.

Transfer the potatoes and carrots to a medium mixing bowl. Add the chick-peas, soy milk, parsley, garlic, scallions, dill weed, pepper, and salt and mash the ingredients together with the back of a spoon or potato masher. (You can also purée the mixture in a blender.) Transfer to a serving bowl and serve warm.

YIELD: 4 SERVINGS

Veggie Bran Raisin Muffins

These delightfully moist muffins make a healthful afternoon snack or light breakfast on the run. They are lowfat, high in fiber, and fortified with carrots and zucchini.

$^{1}/_{2}$ cup orange juice

$^{1}/_{2}$ cup canola oil

$^{1}/_{4}$ cup dark molasses

1 cup brown sugar

2 large eggs, beaten

1 cup wheat bran (unprocessed)

1 cup unbleached all-purpose flour

1 tablespoon baking powder

1 teaspoon salt

1 teaspoon ground allspice

1 teaspoon ground nutmeg

1 cup shredded zucchini

1 cup shredded carrots

$^{1}/_{2}$ cup raisins

$^{1}/_{4}$ cup roasted sunflower seeds (unsalted)

Preheat the oven to 375 degrees F.

In a large mixing bowl combine the juice, oil, molasses, sugar, and eggs; whisk until the batter is creamy. In a separate bowl combine the bran, flour, baking powder, salt, allspice, and nutmeg. Fold into the liquid ingredients, forming a batter. Gently fold in the zucchini, carrots, and raisins.

Pour the batter into a lightly greased muffin tin. Sprinkle the sunflower seeds evenly over the muffins. Place in the oven and bake for about 20 minutes, until a toothpick inserted in the center comes out clean. Remove from the heat and let cool for about 10 minutes before serving.

YIELD: 10 MUFFINS

Banana-Blueberry Bran Bread

This sweet bread is so moist and delicious it could be called "pudding bread." Bananas and blueberries complement each other wonderfully.

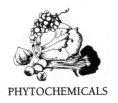

PHYTOCHEMICALS

$^1/_2$ cup canola oil

$^1/_2$ cup applesauce

$^1/_2$ cup lowfat milk

1 cup brown sugar

1 large egg plus 1 egg white

2 cups mashed ripe bananas (about 4 bananas)

$1^1/_2$ cups blueberries

1 cup diced walnuts

$1^1/_2$ cups unbleached all-purpose flour

1 cup wheat bran (unprocessed)

2 teaspoons baking powder

$1^1/_2$ teaspoons ground cinnamon

$^1/_2$ teaspoon salt

Preheat the oven to 375 degrees F.

In a mixing bowl whisk together the oil, applesauce, milk, sugar, and eggs until the batter is creamy. Blend in the mashed bananas, blueberries, and walnuts.

Mix the flour, wheat bran, baking powder, cinnamon, and salt in a separate bowl. Gently fold the dry ingredients into the wet batter. Spoon the batter into two lightly greased 8-inch-by-4-inch loaf pans and bake for 50 to 55 minutes, until a toothpick inserted in the center comes out clean.

Let cool for about 10 minutes on a rack before serving.

YIELD: 2 LOAVES

Pumpkin Fruit Pancakes
with Oat Bran

ANTIOXIDANTS

HEART HEALTHY

Pumpkin and apples lend a flavorful twist to these fiber-rich pancakes. These pancakes make a great Sunday brunch entrée.

1/2 cup all-purpose wheat flour
1/2 cup whole wheat flour
1/2 cup oat or wheat bran
1/3 cup brown sugar
2 teaspoons baking powder
1/2 teaspoon salt
1/2 teaspoon ground nutmeg
1 large egg plus 1 large egg white, beaten
1 1/2 cups soy milk or buttermilk
1 cup mashed pumpkin
2 apples or pears, chopped

Combine the flours, bran, sugar, baking powder, salt, and nutmeg in a medium mixing bowl. In a separate bowl, whisk together the eggs, soy milk or buttermilk, pumpkin, and apples. Fold the liquid batter into the dry ingredients and blend until fully incorporated.

Preheat a lightly greased griddle or skillet over medium heat. Ladle about 1/2 cup of the batter onto the griddle, forming a pancake about 6 inches wide. Cook the pancake for 3 to 4 minutes until the edges begin to brown, then flip. After flipping, press down gently on the pancake with a wide spatula. Continue cooking until the pancake is golden brown. Remove to a warm plate and repeat the process with the remaining batter.

Serve the pancakes with maple syrup.

YIELD: 8 PANCAKES

HELPFUL HINT

If you prefer a thinner pancake, add up to $1/3$ cup more milk to the batter.

Apple Berry Cake

HEART HEALTHY

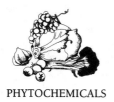

PHYTOCHEMICALS

Diced apples and berries add flavor and nutrients to a variety of cakes and muffins.

1/2 cup orange juice
1/2 cup canola oil
1 cup brown sugar
1/2 cup granulated sugar
2 large eggs
4 cups diced apples
1 1/2 cups fresh raspberries
2 cups all-purpose flour
1 cup whole-wheat flour
1 tablespoon baking powder
1 teaspoon salt
1 teaspoon ground nutmeg
1 teaspoon ground cinnamon
1 cup diced walnuts or pecans
1/4 cup rolled oatmeal

Preheat the oven to 350 degrees F.

In a large mixing bowl blend together the orange juice, oil, brown sugar, and granulated sugar until fully incorporated. Beat in the eggs until creamy. Fold in the apples and raspberries.

In a separate medium mixing bowl combine the flour, baking powder, salt, nutmeg, and cinnamon. Fold the dry mixture into the wet batter. Fold in the nuts.

Pour the batter into a 9-inch round cake pan (sprayed with vegetable oil). Sprinkle with oatmeal. Place the pan on the middle rack in the oven and bake for 50 to 55 minutes, until a toothpick inserted in the center comes out clean. Set on a rack to cool for 20 to 30 minutes.

YIELD: 8 TO 10 SERVINGS

Pillar 3

TREASURES OF THE HEART:
Secrets of Lowfat,
Low-Cholesterol Cooking

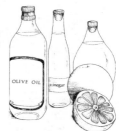

IT SEEMS THAT EVERY DAY WE ARE INUNDATED WITH THE latest revelations about fat, cholesterol, and miracle diets. There are all kinds of fats in the news—body fat, saturated and unsaturated fat, trans fat, lowfat, and fake fat—not to mention the garden varieties of good, bad, and dietary cholesterol. Supermarket aisles bombard us with products screaming "lowfat" or "fat-free," and we voraciously gobble up fat-reduced cookies, ice cream, potato chips, and sundry snacks. Diet cookbooks dominate the bestseller lists, while celebrities unveil their super weight-loss strategies.

Fat, fat, fat. It's on the minds (and sides) of almost everyone. Unfortunately, this elevated level of fat-consciousness has not translated into a culture of healthy lifestyles. Recent surveys have estimated that over one-half of all Americans are considered over-weight—and many are veering toward obesity. We have dipped into the cookie jar and raided the refrigerator one too many times—and the gatekeeper, our willpower, has fallen asleep. It's not just sweets—according to one survey, three of the fastest-growing foods are hamburgers, french fries, and chicken nuggets.

DAZED AND CONFUSED

The expanding girth of the nation's collective waistline is not the only puzzling sign of the times. In spite of this national obsession with fat, cholesterol, and all sorts of dietary crazes, there is a great deal of confusion simmering beneath the surface. What really qualifies as a healthy—or unhealthy—diet? Most people are aware of the long-term dangers posed by eating foods high in fat and cholesterol, but beyond this basic understanding the picture gets murky. When it comes to dietary matters, familiarity does not always breed understanding.

For instance, there is a plethora of questions about the nature of fat itself. Which is healthier, margarine or butter? Is chicken a leaner choice than red meat? Does a glass of 2 percent milk really contain the equivalent fat of three strips of greasy bacon? If olive oil is good for you, is more better? Should you drench your salad in olive oil? If there is a "good" kind of cholesterol, which food contains it? What are *trans fatty acids*? Can you eat as many lowfat cookies as you want and not gain weight?

When the topic of fat comes up, a blizzard of questions (and opinions) abound. Trying to understand a good diet's connection to good health is like riding a merry-go-round, only at times it ain't so merry.

In the past fifty years the world of nutritional science has made great strides in understanding the link between dietary fat, cholesterol, and chronic disease. It is widely known that the typical high-fat, meat-based diet found in Western societies is at the root of many illnesses. Unfortunately, the drumbeat of health communiqués and attention-grabbing headlines has confused people and often raises more questions. To further complicate matters, it seems everyone can recite at least one exception. There's the inevitable ninety-year-old friend who cooks with butter, loves to eat jumbo eggs, smokes a pack of cigarettes every day, and quaffs a pint of whiskey after dinner.

There is a bottom line to this discussion: heart disease and cancer are the nation's top two killer diseases. Every year heart disease and cancer rob millions of Americans of their ability to enjoy the prime years of their life. The typical Western diet—high in saturated fat and cholesterol and short on fiber, antioxidants, and phytochemicals—has been fingered as a major risk factor in the development of heart disease, certain cancers, and other chronic diseases.

There is little doubt that our diet plays a major role in both quantity and quality of life. Despite the inevitable aberrations, diet and longevity go hand in hand. Cut to the chase: a grandparent's enjoyment of his or her grandchildren may be directly linked to life-long eating habits. The kind of dietary lifestyle may determine whether one spends the prime-time years strolling on a golf course or cultivating a garden—or lying on a couch or hospital bed.

When it comes to making food choices and dietary decisions, the stakes are high. The issue begs for more than a vague understanding or placing credence in simplistic anecdotes. Learning about the risks posed by dietary fat and cholesterol may be as important as coming to grips with the dangers posed by cigarettes and tobacco. It is well known that maintaining a heavy smoking habit is akin to a death wish. Dietary fat may be the next Public Enemy Number One.

THE JIG IS UP: RECOGNIZING THE TRUTH ABOUT FAT AND CHOLESTEROL

There is clear and overwhelming evidence that a diet rich in saturated fat and cholesterol can dramatically increase the risk of heart disease, the nation's number-one killer. Also known as coronary

FACTS ON FAT

- Fats are also called lipids. All fats are composed of varying amounts of fatty acids, the building blocks of fat. Cholesterol is one type of fat.

- Fats contain nine calories per gram, over twice the amount found in protein or complex carbohydrates. Excess calories are stored as body fat.

- The three most common types of fatty acids in foods are saturated fat, monounsaturated fat, and polyunsaturated fat. Dietary fats contain varying proportions of each type of fatty acid. For example, butter contains about 70 percent saturated fat and is classified as a saturated fat. Canola oil contains 60 percent monounsaturated fats and is classified as such.

- A fourth type of fat, called trans fatty acid, is a vegetable oil that has been chemically altered ("hydrogenated") to exhibit a semisolid texture. In simple terms, a liquid unsaturated fat is engineered to become more saturated and solid. Margarine is a prime example of a food product containing "partially hydrogenated vegetable oil," or trans fatty acids.

artery disease, heart disease prevents millions of Americans every year from pursuing a healthy and rewarding life. Furthermore, high-fat diets have been associated with an increased risk of obesity, diabetes, stroke, and certain cancers. In other words, a high-fat, meat-based diet will adversely impact millions of people every year by causing chronic degenerative diseases.

The surplus of dietary fat and cholesterol is not the only problem. The typical diet of meat and potatoes (or chicken swimming in gravy) also lacks many of the life-promoting, disease-fighting substances found in a healthful plant-based diet. A week's meal plan filled with buttered toast, bacon, ham and cheese sandwiches, mayonnaise dressings, hamburgers, cream soups, marbled steaks, sausages, hot dogs, and pie à la mode leaves little room for nutrient-dense vegetables, grains, beans, and fruits. Not only does the typical meat- or chicken-based diet contribute to chronic disease, it crowds out all those beneficial antioxidants, phyto-nutrients, fiber, and complex carbohydrates. That's not a double whammy, it's a *multiple* whammy!

For years it has been generally known that fat and cholesterol are major roadblocks in the highway to a healthy life. To thor-oughly understand and appreciate how a diet high in fat and cho-lesterol can increase the risk of disease, contribute to a lesser quality of life, and steer life down a dead-end road, one must de-construct the process step by step. Along the way it will be possi-ble to make better choices about the food you eat. You've heard it thousands of times, but the cliché rings true: you are what you eat.

FIRST, AN IN-DEPTH LOOK AT CHOLESTEROL

The term *cholesterol* has been indelibly stamped into the minds of most Americans. Cholesterol has a high "Q-rating," like certain soft drinks and fast-food chains. There is a general agreement that too much cholesterol circulating in the body (a high cholesterol count) is not a good omen. Most people know that cholesterol is found exclusively in foods of animal origin (such as meat, chicken, butter, eggs, shellfish, and so forth). On the other hand, vegetables, fruits, grains, beans—actually, all plant foods—are nat-urally free of cholesterol.

Beyond this point, the public's understanding of cholesterol grows dim. What exactly is cholesterol, this vilified bane to the healthy heart? Cholesterol is a kind of fat, specifically a white, waxy fatty substance. Cholesterol is naturally produced in every-one's body by the liver and, believe it or not, actually plays a vital role in bodily functions. Among many things, cholesterol helps in the production of hormones, assists in the building of cell walls, and aids in the digestion and absorption of dietary fat. The liver does a commendable job in manufacturing all of the cholesterol our bodies need; therefore, there is never a requirement to eat foods that contain cholesterol.

The trouble begins when there is too much cholesterol circulating in the bloodstream of our body. Over time the excess cholesterol in the blood (called serum cholesterol) begins to cling to the inside walls of the blood vessels and arteries leading to and from the heart. As cholesterol continues to accumulate in the bloodstream, a residue called *plaque* forms inside the arteries. This is the crux of the problem. The cholesterol-laden plaque eventually gums up and clogs the arteries. The obstructed passageways become narrower and narrower and can lead to arteriosclerosis, a form of heart disease. If the clogged artery leads to the heart, the result can be a heart attack. If the clogged artery blocks the blood flowing to the brain, a stroke can occur.

To visualize how an artery becomes blocked by cholesterol, think of the drain pipes beneath your kitchen sink. When you clean your dirty plates, food waste goes down the drain. As time goes by, remnants of the waste stick and cling to the inside walls of the drain pipes. The passage narrows, liquids cease to drain freely, and eventually the pipes become clogged. The sink backs up and it's time to get the plunger. Just as the drains beneath your sink become obstructed over time (not all at once), the arteries in our bodies can become clogged over the course of a lifetime of unhealthy eating habits. (When a doctor tries to unplug or unclog a choked artery, the procedure is called angioplasty.)

THE GOOD, THE BAD, AND THE UGLY

So, cholesterol is a serious matter. Generally speaking, a high level of cholesterol in the bloodstream is a cardinal risk factor for heart disease and stroke. A high cholesterol reading is one signal that trouble may be brewing. By itself, the overall cholesterol count depicts a broad picture and requires further examination. There is more than one type of cholesterol circulating in the body and, surprisingly, not all of the blood cholesterol is considered bad for our health.

There are two prominent types of blood cholesterol to consider: high density lipoproteins, also called HDL, or "good cholesterol," and low-density lipoproteins, also called LDL, or "bad cholesterol." (To a lesser extent there is a third type called very-low-density lipoproteins, or VLDL.) In scientific terms, cholesterol is transported in the bloodstream by these lipoproteins. The lipoproteins wrap around the cholesterol like a blanket and carry the fatty substances throughout the body. To fully grasp the significance of cholesterol, it is important to understand the differences between "good" HDL and "bad" LDL.

Low-density lipoproteins supply the arteries with cholesterol and can lead to a dangerous plaque buildup. Consequently, LDL is known as bad cholesterol (think "L for *lethal*"). An abundance of LDL will enable plaque to lodge in the arteries and dramatically increase the risk of heart attack or stroke. Low-density lipoproteins are heavy with cholesterol baggage and light with protein.

High-density lipoproteins circulating in the bloodstream actually pluck the bad cholesterol off the artery walls and flush it back to the liver for excretion. (This process is called "reverse cholesterol transport.") In the process, HDL helps to prevent the harmful plaque from building up in the arteries. As a result, HDL is known as good cholesterol (think "H for *healthy*"). High-density lipoproteins are rich in protein and light on cholesterol. Displaying a low level of good cholesterol is considered to be a risk factor for heart disease.

Although our bodies manufacture both good and bad kinds of cholesterol, about 70 to 75 percent is bad cholesterol and only 25 percent is good. Fortunately, there are ways to increase the good cholesterol and decrease the bad (and vice versa). The goal of a heart-smart lifestyle is not only to decrease overall cholesterol, but to increase the production of good cholesterol and decrease the production of (or flush out) bad cholesterol. (See Table 3.1.)

The goal of a heart-smart lifestyle is not only to decrease overall cholesterol, but to increase the production of good cholesterol and decrease the production of (or flush out) bad cholesterol.

TABLE 3.1
Making Sense of Dietary Fats

Dietary Fat	Sources	Characteristics	Effects on Cholesterol
Saturated Fats	Animal foods, such as butter, lard, marbled meats, hamburger, poultry skin, cream, and cheese. Also, coconut and palm oil.	Solid at room temperature	Elevate the "bad" cholesterol circulating in the body and lead to clogged arteries.
Monounsaturated Fats	Olive oil, canola oil, peanut oil, and avocados.	Liquid at room temperature	Decrease bad cholesterol and increase good cholesterol.
Polyunsaturated Fats	Corn oil, safflower oil, sesame oil, and fish oils (omega-3 fats).	Liquid at room temperature	May decrease both bad and good types of cholesterol.
Trans Fats	Margarines, vegetable shortening, and processed foods containing partially hydrogenated vegetable oils.	Semisolid at room temperature	May increase bad cholesterol levels and decrease good cholesterol.

WHAT ABOUT DIETARY CHOLESTEROL?

Up to this point, the discussion has focused on the two main types of cholesterol circulating in our bloodstreams. There is another kind of cholesterol to be reckoned with: *dietary cholesterol*. This type of cholesterol is found exclusively in animal foods—meat, chicken, bacon, eggs, dairy products, etc. Another key point: dietary cholesterol tends to travel with saturated fat, another health nemesis. (As I mentioned earlier, plant foods contain zero cholesterol. Apples, broccoli, rice, pasta, beans, nuts—the whole check-list of plant-based foods—are totally free of cholesterol.)

It would be logical to blame high serum cholesterol levels (and heart disease) on diets based on cholesterol-rich animal foods. After all, the average American diet contains from 400 to 600 milligrams of cholesterol per day, an amount far higher than the recommended level of 300 milligrams. It *seems* like a logical theory: reduce the amount of cholesterol in your diet, and blood cholesterol levels will also drop.

But the relationship between dietary cholesterol and your body's cholesterol level is not quite that simple. Research has borne out that the cholesterol derived from a diet of hamburgers, chicken, shrimp, milk, and so forth does not necessarily raise blood cholesterol levels in everyone. It seems that some people compensate by ceasing to manufacture their own cholesterol—their livers slow down the production line. Or perhaps their bodies compensate by excreting the excess cholesterol. Either way, the cholesterol in food may not be directly linked to the cholesterol in your body. It turns out that dietary cholesterol may not be the culprit many people thought it was.

Is dietary cholesterol off the hook? Does this realization provide more ammunition for naysayers and skeptics? Not quite. Linking the food we eat to cholesterol and heart disease has been the subject of much research, debate, and conjecture. Remember, dietary cholesterol travels with saturated fat. Foods high in cholesterol also tend to be rich in saturated fat. For years researchers focused on dietary cholesterol while saturated fats stood in the shadows.

Where there's smoke, there's fire. It turns out that the saturated fat in the foods we eat may raise the level of bad cholesterol in our bodies, depress the good cholesterol, and initiate a domino effect that leads to heart disease. The saturated fat—more than the dietary cholesterol—has a greater negative impact on the condition of the heart. Dietary fat not only adds to your body weight, it may threaten your health.

The saturated fat—more than the dietary cholesterol—has a greater negative impact on the condition of the heart.

CONTROLLING YOUR CHOLESTEROL: TWELVE POINTS WORTH PONDERING

1. Exercising regularly can increase the level of good cholesterol.

2. Cooking with monounsaturated fats (such as olive oil and canola oil) can increase the protective good cholesterol and decrease the bad cholesterol.

3. Losing weight has been shown to increase the level of good cholesterol. Excess body weight tends to raise bad cholesterol and suppress good cholesterol.

4. Foods rich in soluble fiber (such beans, apples, oatmeal, oat bran) may lower total cholesterol levels while increasing good cholesterol. (See Pillar 2: Discover the Goodness of Fiber.)

5. Saturated fats increase the production of bad cholesterol. Reducing consumption of foods high in saturated fat (such as butter, red meat, bacon fat, lard, tropical oils, and heavy cream) can lower bad cholesterol.

6. Limit the intake of processed foods containing trans fats (such as margarine, baked goods, and snacks). Trans fats may increase the production of bad cholesterol.

7. Don't smoke. If you do smoke, quit. Aside from causing lung damage, smoking has been shown to increase overall cholesterol and decrease the production of good cholesterol.

8. Cut back on foods rich in dietary cholesterol. Although saturated fat has a greater effect on serum cholesterol levels, dietary cholesterol travels with saturated fat.

9. Plant-based foods rich in antioxidant nutrients may thwart the oxidation of LDL and prevent plaque from forming. (For plaque to form in the arteries, cholesterol must undergo an oxidation process fueled by unstable free radicals.) Antioxidants are found in dark leafy greens, orange and yellow fruits and vegetables, and citrus fruits. (For more on antioxidants, turn to Pillar 1: Unleash the Power of Antioxidants.)

10. When you see a commercial for "antacid relief," think "fatty acid" relief. Fatty foods not only increase blood cholesterol levels and add to body fat, they are high in acids and hard to digest. It's the fatty acids and amino acids that cause indigestion, not the herbs or spices.

11. Remember that animal proteins may also raise cholesterol, so shifting from red meat to chicken is not considered an option in the effort to reduce your cholesterol count.

12. Remember that animal foods are made of saturated fat and protein and little else. Ground beef is 60 to 80 percent fat, chicken is 25 to 50 percent fat, and lean beef is still 35 to 40 percent fat. Even when you trim the fat off of steaks or chicken, you are still left with protein and dietary fat—and no fiber or energy-supplying complex carbohydrates. In addition, so-called "lowfat" 2 percent milk derives over 20 percent of calories from fat.

THE PLOT THICKENS: DIETARY FAT ENTERS THE EQUATION

Before we tackle the concept of saturated fat, it is necessary to expound upon the diverse range of fats, also known as *lipids*. There's a lot about fat to decipher. In addition to saturated fat, there is monounsaturated fat, polyunsaturated fat, trans fat, and synthetic or "fake" fat. And, of course, there's body fat, where excess dietary fat gets deposited and stored. Cholesterol is another type of fat. All fats are made of combinations of fatty acids (just as proteins are constructed of amino acids).

It is no secret that the average American diet contains far too much fat. Fat calories make up about 40 percent of the foods we eat—way above the 30 percent of calories recommended by most nutritionists. For optimal health, some renowned experts in the field (such as Dr. Dean Ornish and Dr. John McDougall) urge that fat calories be restricted to about *10 percent* of total calories, which would clearly require a radical change in the way most people eat.

Fat appears in a variety of guises throughout the food chain. Dietary fat lends a smooth texture to cream sauces and spreads (like mayonnaise and hollandaise). Fat gives a silky consistency to decadent desserts (custard, chocolate mousse, and ice cream). In snack foods and candy, fat teams up with sodium and sugar to satisfy our primordial cravings for sweet and salty tastes. Meat eaters savor "marbled" steak for its juiciness (marbling refers to the streaks of fat woven throughout the meat). From lobster bisque and fettuccine Alfredo to french fries, potato chips, doughnuts, and buttery pound cake, fat is in all of the foods we love to eat.

Nutritionists are quick to point out that not all dietary fat should be avoided. Fat is an essential nutrient and performs myriad tasks; it supplies energy, regulates metabolism, and assists in forming cell membranes. Body fat keeps us warm in cold weather. However, just one tablespoon of fat a day would meet our daily needs. The average Western diet contains far more than one tablespoon a day of fat.

WHAT BECOMES OF ALL THE EXCESS DIETARY FAT?

It becomes body fat, of course. The surplus of fat in our diet gets stored as body fat and ultimately arrives on our thighs, chins, waistlines, and other familiar places. Leftover calories from protein and carbohydrates also get stored as body fat. This accumulated fat is not burned off until carbohydrates, the main source of energy, are depleted. (Another way to burn off body fat is to exercise aerobically for at least twenty minutes a day.)

Given our high consumption of dietary fat, it is not surprising that most people in this country are overweight. In simplistic terms, we gain weight and develop layers of fatty tissue because there is a surplus of calories in the typical animal-based diet. The "energy in" part of the equation exceeds the "energy out," or the calories used up. Of course, other factors contribute to the ballooning body shapes. Genetics, metabolism, frequency of exercise, work environment, and lifestyle habits all affect our body size and shape. Still, the fat-laden diet is the major determinant. Fat begets fat.

An overweight population is not the only consequence of society's high fat intake. The larger problem is that the excessive fat in the Western diet has been implicated as a major risk factor in a range of diseases. Specifically, the kind and amount of fat you consume may well determine whether you are steering your body toward a collision with heart disease, stroke, or cancer. The repercussions to your long-term health are indeed profound.

ALL FATS ARE NOT CREATED EQUAL

A stick of butter, a cup of olive oil, a tub of margarine, and lard from beef may all be related but they are not interchangeable. When it comes to matters of health and nutrition there are big differences in the types of fat in one's diet. For example, olive oil (which is high in monounsaturated fats) may actually offer *protection* against cholesterol buildup and heart disease. The saturated fat found in red meat, lard, and butter exhibits a detrimental effect on overall health. Saturated fat raises the level of bad cholesterol and contributes to heart disease.

AN IN-DEPTH LOOK AT DIETARY FATS

Although the fatty acids are all members of the same family, the ramifications associated with each type of fat vary significantly.

Saturated Fats

Saturated fats are found mostly in animal foods. Butter, lard, cheese, marbled red meat, chicken, eggs, whole milk, and ice cream all contain saturated fat. There are a few plant foods, such as coconut oil and palm oil, also on the list. It is easy to spot a saturated fat: as a rule, saturated fats are solid at room temperature.

When it comes to matters of the heart, saturated fats are "the bad guys." There is strong evidence to suggest that saturated fat elevates the level of bad cholesterol circulating in our bodies (and increases the risk of heart disease). Studies have shown that saturated fat may stimulate our livers to produce more bad cholesterol or impair our body's ability to flush out the bad cholesterol already in our bloodstream. Whatever the scenario, a diet high in saturated fat can lead to high cholesterol, plaque buildup, and gummed-up arteries.

Monounsaturated Fats

Monounsaturated fats are prevalent in plant foods and vegetable oils. Olive oil, canola oil, and peanut oil are good sources of unsaturated fats. As a general rule, monounsaturated fats are liquid at room temperature.

Monounsaturated fats are "the good guys." There is good reason to believe that monounsaturated fats may actually decrease the artery-clogging bad cholesterol in the blood and increase the amount of good cholesterol. Mediterranean and Asian populations, whose diets are largely based on plant foods and monounsaturated vegetable oils, exhibit lower rates of heart disease and certain cancers. Experts believe that monounsaturated fats may be a chief reason why those populations avoid the scourges associated with Western diets rich in saturated fats.

Polyunsaturated Fats

Polyunsaturated fats are prevalent in plant foods, vegetable oils, and fish oils. Sunflower oil, safflower oil, and corn oil are good sources of polyunsaturated fats. Like monounsaturated fats, poly-unsaturated fats tend to be liquid at room temperature.

Polyunsaturated fats offer a bag of mixed messages; these fats are believed to reduce *both* the good *and* the bad kinds of cholesterol. Furthermore, most margarines are made by partially hydrogenating (adding hydrogen to) polyunsaturated fats. This process transforms a liquid fat into a semisolid substance and creates a synthetic "trans fat," a cross between a saturated fat and an unsaturated fat. Trans fats have also been implicated in elevating bad cholesterol.

THE LETHAL LINK BETWEEN SATURATED FAT, CHOLESTEROL, AND HEART DISEASE

The body of scientific research devoted to diet and heart disease is of mammoth proportions and can be overwhelming. There is an abundance of literature that blames saturated fat for multiple harms, including raising the risk of heart disease. In an attempt to clarify matters, here are some key points to ponder.

• A meat-based diet tends to contain large amounts of saturated fat and dietary cholesterol, two leading factors in heart disease and other chronic ailments.

• Saturated fat travels hand in hand with dietary cholesterol. Both substances may be responsible for raising serum cholesterol levels.

• A plant-based diet with mainly monounsaturated fats (such as olive oil) can lead to a decreased risk of heart disease.

• One more strike against excessive consumption of red meat and chicken: there is growing reason to suspect that diets high in animal proteins may also raise cholesterol levels.

• Cutting back on saturated fat can significantly reduce the risk of heart attack or stroke.

In the long run, there is much to gain from reducing consumption of foods high in saturated fats (animal foods) and shifting to a plant-based diet that includes monounsaturated fats.

AN IN-DEPTH LOOK AT TRANS FATS

When the perils of saturated fat first came to the light in the mid-1950s, many people gave up butter and lard and started using margarine, the less expensive spread made with hydrogenated vegetable oils. Margarine contains less saturated fat than solid butter but has more fat than unsaturated liquid vegetable oils have. For years margarine was considered a healthy and economical alternative to butter, animal fats, and other saturated fats.

Unfortunately, the happy story of margarine takes a disturbing twist. To make margarine, vegetable oils are partially hydrogenated. The "good" unsaturated fats are transformed into saturated fats. The process creates a shadowy, chemically altered substance called trans fats. Generally speaking, the more solid the vegetable oil, the more trans fats the product contains. (A stick of firm margarine has more trans fats than soft margarine sold in a tub.)

Trans fats are scientifically altered fats made by adding hydrogen to vegetable oils. The process, called *hydrogenation*, makes the fat semisolid at room temperature, makes it less prone to rancidity, and extends the shelf life. Margarine and vegetable shortenings are partially hydrogenated vegetable oils. There are also countless supermarket foods that contain partially hydrogenated oils. Examples include crackers, cookies, potato chips, salad dressings, peanut butter, and baked goods.

WILL TRANS FATTY ACID BECOME THE FRANKENSTEIN OF FAT?

There is emerging evidence to support the charge that the synthesized trans fats may not only raise bad cholesterol levels but

The goal of a healthful diet is to cut back on both saturated fats and trans fatty acids and to seek out healthful alternatives. Here are tasty ways to avoid both butter and margarine.

THE BUTTER OR MARGARINE "NON-DEBATE"

- Sauté with vegetable oils such as canola oil and olive oil instead of margarine or butter.
- Dip warm bread into a small dish of olive oil as the Italians do. (Skip the butter and margarine.)
- On toast or muffins, spread jam, not butter or margarine.
- Shop for quality fresh-baked bread that tastes great on its own and does not require excessive embellishment.
- Read the labels of cookies, crackers, and snack foods and moderate your consumption of foods listing partially hydrogenated vegetable oils.
- On corn, use lime for basting instead of butter or margarine.
- Season potatoes and vegetables with lemon juice, herbs, or spices, not margarine or butter.
- Limit the amount of fried foods in your diet—especially taco shells, doughnuts, chicken nuggets, and french fries that have been fried in vegetable shortening or lard.
- Choose tub margarine or "liquid squeeze" margarine over stick margarine. Choose "light" margarine over full-fat varieties. (The more liquid the fat at room temperature, the less saturated it is.)
- Choose baking recipes that call for vegetable oil, not butter, shortening, or margarine.
- Read the labels of processed foods (cereals, cookies, dressings) and whenever possible choose brands that do not include partially hydrogenated vegetable oils.

also suppress good cholesterol—a double blow to your heart. Healthy unsaturated fats have been transformed into portentous cholesterol-raising fats. Margarine, it turns out, may be worse for your heart than butter.

Is this a genuine risk or false alarm? Some experts argue that foods like margarine are used in such small portions that the effect on cholesterol levels is minimal. On the other hand, partially hydrogenated vegetable oils are widely used in the nation's food supply. Fast-food restaurants use copious amounts of vegetable shortening to fry everything from french fries, taco shells, and fried haddock to doughnuts and apple turnovers. Furthermore, the amount of trans fats in a product is not required to be listed on food nutrition labels, so it is difficult to gauge the amount of trans fats in processed foods.

One thing is certain: when the nation's overall fat consumption shifts from saturated fats to trans fats, there is no real health gain. Until more is known about the long-term effects of trans fat, the best advice is to treat margarine and vegetable shortening like any other saturated fat and *use them sparingly*.

One thing is certain: when the nation's overall fat consumption shifts from saturated fats to trans fats, there is no real health gain. Until more is known about the long-term effects of trans fat, the best advice is to treat margarine and vegetable shortening like any other saturated fat and use them sparingly.

THE ANIMAL PROTEIN–CHOLESTEROL CONNECTION

As if the saturated fat found in animal foods were not bad enough, recent studies have implied that animal protein may also raise blood cholesterol levels—even in the absence of dietary cholesterol. Taken another way, when the so-called "complete" proteins found in animal foods (meat, chicken, and dairy products) are replaced in the diet with plant proteins (found in soy foods, beans), the cholesterol level drops. Amino acids in meat-based foods may hinder the body's ability to flush out "bad" cholesterol. In the quest for a healthy life, this is yet another reason to consider shifting from a meat-based diet to a plant-based diet. It doesn't help that animal protein travels with saturated fat and dietary cholesterol. (For more on protein, turn to Pillar 4: Exploding the Protein Myths.)

There is still much to be learned about the tangled web of saturated fat, trans fats, cholesterol, and heart disease. Additionally, there are other lifestyle factors at work. Family history, blood pressure, smoking habits, and a sedentary (or active) lifestyle all play significant roles in the health of the heart. The one factor we can control is diet, and reducing consumption of foods high in saturated fats is one giant step on the path to a healthy lifestyle.

TWENTY WAYS TO REDUCE THE FAT AND CHOLESTEROL IN YOUR DIET

A healthful diet can significantly decrease the risk of heart attack or stroke. A 10 to 15 percent reduction in blood cholesterol levels can reduce the risk of coronary heart disease by 20 to 30 percent.

Here are twenty ways to reduce the fat and cholesterol in your diet while enriching your overall health. Some are specific actions; others are offered as general rules (or, food for thought, if you will).

1. Shift from a meat-based diet to a plant-based diet. Eat more vegetables, grains, pastas, and beans and fewer animal foods high in saturated fat.

2. Designate at least one day a week to "go meatless." Then designate two days, then three days, and so forth. Start now.

3. Read the labels of processed foods and avoid products containing beef lard, beef fat, chicken fat, or tropical oils. Beef bouillon cubes are a good example of products to avoid.

4. Drink skim milk or 1 percent milk. Blend in soy milk with dairy milk (or switch to soy milk altogether).

5. Avoid non-dairy creamers containing tropical oils or partially hydrogenated vegetable oils.

6. Cook with cheese made from lowfat or part skim milk. Substitute lowfat yogurt for sour cream or cream cheese in dip recipes.

7. Limit your consumption of eggs to two or fewer per week.

8. In baking recipes, remove half of the egg yolks (but keep the egg whites) called for in the recipe.

9. Sauté with canola oil instead of butter, shortening, or margarine.

10. Commercial salad dressings often contain too much fat, sugar, monosodium glutamate, sodium, and other additives. Try a homemade vinaigrette made with olive oil or canola oil, vinegar, and herbs.

11. Avoid fried foods on restaurant and diner menus. French fries, potato wedges, chicken wings, doughnuts, fried haddock, and fish and chips are kingpins of fat.

12. Avoid fast-food standards that are notoriously high in fat. Fish and chicken sandwiches, processed chicken nuggets, onion rings, hash browns, and apple or cherry turnovers are dripping with fat.

13. Eat foods that are high in soluble fibers (pectin, guar, psyllium) such as oatmeal, oat bran bread, beans, and apples. Soluble fiber may lower blood cholesterol levels.

14. Serve salsa in place of dips made with full-fat sour cream (such as French onion dip).

15. Treat yourself to lowfat ice cream or yogurt, sorbet, or frozen fruit ices. Save the premium ice creams for special occasions.

16. Avoid eating meals with fatty cream sauces. Examples include fettuccine Alfredo, casseroles made with cream of mushroom soup, seafood Newburg, and cream bisques.

17. Whenever you see the term *streusel topping*, think "fat and sugar."

18. Choose a baked potato over french fries; mustard over mayonnaise; and vinaigrette over creamy dressings like Thousand Island or creamy Italian.

19. Serve pasta with a red sauce, not white sauce. Choose Manhattan clam chowder (made with a tomato broth) over New England clam chowder (made with cream).

20. Use cheese as a garnish (sparingly), not as a main ingredient. Avoid cheese-dominated dishes such as lasagna, cheese sauce, cheese soup, and quiche.

THE FAKERY BEHIND FAKE FATS

Most people have heard of olestra by now, the synthetic fat substitute with zero calories. Apparently it tastes and cooks like real fat and has a fatty feel in the mouth. Olestra, which is also known by its trade name, "Olean," is intended to replace the fat used in processing potato chips, tortilla chips, french fries, crackers, and other snack foods. Olestra is one of many fat-free additives beginning to show up in processed foods. (Other brands of fake fats include Appetize and Simplesse.)

Although fake fats do not add on the calories, neither are they panaceas for poor eating habits. If anything, studies have shown that people will make up the calories elsewhere (most likely by eating *more* chips). Some believe that fake fats will only stimulate demand for foods with the real thing. In addition, fake fats may reduce the absorption of carotenoids and fat-soluble vitamins, an effect that could deprive people of essential disease-fighting

TABLE 3.2

Out with the Old, in with the New

Yesterday's Choice	The Problem	Healthy Alternatives
Pasta Alfredo	Heavy with cream, eggs, butter, and cheese.	Choose a meatless tomato sauce such as marinara, spicy arrabbiata, or Neapolitan sauce.
Hollandaise and béarnaise	Sauces oozing with butter, egg yolks, and oil.	Tomato salsa, fruit salsa, guacamole, or piquant Creole sauce.
Cheese fondue	Made with cream, butter, and shredded cheese.	Bean dips such as hummus or black bean purée.
Butter sauces	Swimming in fat. Typical ½ cup serving contains a whopping 800 calories and 100 grams of fat.	Sofrito, a mix of onion, peppers, tomatoes, garlic, and cilantro. Or red sauces or Creole sauce.
Pancakes or French toast drowned in butter	Why start the day with a fat attack?	Pancake topping of berries, chopped apples, or bananas.
Potatoes topped with sour cream or butter	A good source of complex carbohydrates is ruined with fat.	Serve lowfat yogurt, salsa, black bean sauce, or *raita,* a cucumber sauce.
Gravy	Made with the fatty pan drippings of roast poultry or meats.	Try a vegetable gravy made with vegetable stock.
Fruit with chantilly sauce	Healthy fruit is bombarded with heavy cream and sugar.	Try a squeeze of lime or a dollop of lowfat yogurt sweetened with honey.
Chili con carne	Chili is made with greasy ground meat.	Try a meatless chili with red beans and vegetables.
Corn on the cob slathered with butter or margarine	Why drench fresh corn in fat?	Squeeze fresh lime and sprinkle with cayenne or chili powder.

nutrients. There is also well-publicized anecdotal evidence to suggest that olestra snacks may cause gastric distress and flatulence in some people.

All in all, deciding to eat foods processed with fake fats is a personal choice, but definitely not a healthy choice.

THE HEART-HEALTHY KITCHEN

Here's a revelation: meals that are low in fat and cholesterol do not have to be bland, uninspiring, or served in minuscule portions. In today's enlightened kitchen there is a variety of creative ways to include heart-friendly staples in your diet. Heart-healthy cuisine can be vibrant, satisfying, and bursting with flavors. All that is necessary is a wide assortment of pantry staples, a little creativity, and a willingness to discard an addiction to high-fat ingredients (see Table 3.2). If the taste buds lead the way, the willpower is bound to follow.

This section includes a glossary of ingredients found in the heart-smart pantry. Healthful cooking depends upon a wide assortment of vinegars, cooking wines, monounsaturated oils, citrus fruits, healthful condiments, and lowfat dairy products. In addition, there is a guide to salad greens and lowfat sauces.

Here are a few tips to keep in mind.

Experiment: Explore the growing array of high-flavor, lowfat staples. Flavor your foods with lemons, limes, wine vinegars, cooking wines, mustards, and lowfat yogurt.

Avoid Saturated Fats: Limit the consumption of (or avoid altogether) foods rich in saturated fats and dietary cholesterol. Beef, pork, bacon, cream, butter, and tropical oils top the unwanted list.

Avoid Trans Fats: Limit the consumption of foods containing trans fats. Margarine is a prime example, but there are scores of processed foods listing partially hydrogenated vegetable oils as a main ingredient.

Read the Ingredients: Read the labels of processed foods. Labels boasting "low cholesterol" are not necessarily a healthful choice. Low-cholesterol foods can contain artery-clogging saturated fats or partially hydrogenated vegetable oils.

Read the Nutritional Analysis: Beware of "lowfat" foods based on unrealistic (and deceptive) serving sizes! For example, one 12-ounce package of "lowfat" bacon listed only 25 fat calories *per serving,* but the analysis was based on 24 servings, at *1/2 strip per serving.* Don't be fooled.

Long-Term Effects: Reducing your cholesterol can have life-altering consequences. A 10 to 15 percent reduction in blood cholesterol levels can reduce the risk of heart disease by 20 to 30 percent.

Vim and Vinegar

Vinegar is a true hero in the healthful kitchen. With negligible calories and tart flavors, vinegar enhances a variety of foods without adding an ounce of fat. Vinaigrettes, salad dressings, marinades, and delicate soups and sauces all profit from the deft use of vinegar.

A Cook's Guide to Vinegars

Here is a glossary of vinegars. There is a wider assortment to choose from than you might have expected.

Balsamic Vinegar has a mellow flavor with a hint of tartness and a purplish brown hue. Made from well-aged grape juice, balsamic vinegar is imported from Italy. Balsamic vinegar's distinctive presence makes it easy to reduce the oil in sauces and salad dressings. This vinegar is a must-have staple in the healthy pantry.

Champagne Vinegar has a smooth, mild flavor with a subtle champagne nuance. Reserve this vinegar for special occasions.

Cider Vinegar is a mild, fruity vinegar. Pause and you'll smell a bouquet of tart apples and pears. Cider vinegar makes a good addition to dressings and chutneys.

Flavored Vinegars come in a variety of flavors: raspberry, tarragon, basil, garlic, hot chilies, ginger, and other aromatic varieties. Flavored vinegars are a convenient way to add zest to salad dressings and pasta salads.

Red Wine Vinegar has a mellow tartness and medium body. It is the most versatile and economical of grape vinegars and qualifies as a "workhorse." Use red wine vinegar in salad dressings, chutneys, pasta and potato salads, and vinaigrettes for vegetables.

Rice Vinegar, made from rice wine, has a smooth, almost sweet flavor. It is prevalent in Asian cuisine. Use rice vinegar in stir-fries, salads, and dressings.

Sherry Vinegar, made from dry sherry, is popular in European dressings and salads.

White Wine Vinegar has a mild flavor similar to champagne vinegar. White wine vinegar should not be confused with clear vinegar (which is made from alcohol).

Heart-Healthy Vegetable Oils

Just as there are good fats and bad fats, there are good oils and bad oils. In general, choose vegetable oils that are high in monounsaturated fats and low in saturated fats (such as olive oil and canola oil). Avoid or use sparingly any type of animal fat or tropical oil. Consumption of margarine (which contains semisaturated trans fats) should also be limited.

Keep in mind that the heart-healthy oils (olive oil and canola oil) still contain fat and should be used in moderation. They are good fats but if overused will easily add to your body's storage of fat.

A Cook's Guide to Healthful Cooking Oils
Here is a glossary of the various "good" oils on the market. Each type has a unique flavor and purpose.

Canola Oil, also called rapeseed oil, is a versatile oil high in monounsaturated fats. Canola oil is good for salads, baking, and skillet cooking. (Puritan is a popular brand name.)

Corn Oil is a mildly flavored oil. It is a good staple for basic cooking recipes and salad dressings.

Olive Oil, the treasured oil in Mediterranean cooking, has a rich olive flavor. Olive oil is the best source of monounsaturated fats. There are two basic types available: extra virgin and pure olive oil. Extra virgin is made from the first pressing of olives and has a luscious, desirable taste. Extra virgin is ideal for salad dressings but should not be used for cooking (it has a low smoking point). The next pressing of olives yields "pure" olive oil. Pure olive oil can be used for cooking and salad dressings.

Peanut Oil has a mild nutty flavor and is a good source of monounsaturated fats. Peanut oil is prevalent in Asian cuisine; stir-fried recipes often call for peanut oil.

Safflower Oil has a distinctive flavor and is perhaps too strong for salad dressing. Made from yellow safflower seeds, it is low in saturated fats and high in polyunsaturated fats.

Citrus Juices, Wines, Broths, and Vegetable Juices

While vinegars and oils form the core of many dishes, there is also room in the pantry for lowfat liquids such as citrus juices, dry wines, vegetable broths, and fresh juices.

A Cook's Guide to Lowfat Cooking Liquids

Try experimenting with the different cooking liquids available. Here is a guide suggesting how best to use each one.

Lemon Juice can add a tangy flavor to light pasta and vegetable dishes, grain salads such as tabbouleh, roasted vegetables, broccoli, asparagus, and tossed leafy greens. Lemon juice can also perk up potato soups and chowders. For optimum flavor, squeeze the lemon just before serving.

Lime Juice can be spritzed over black bean dishes, rice and bean salads, salsa, guacamole, and corn on the cob.

Red Wine adds robust flavors to tomato-based sauces (marinara, arrabbiata, Creole, and other meatless red sauces), hearty bean stews, and tomato and vegetable soups. For best results use a dry red wine, not a sweet fruity wine.

Vegetable and *Fruit Juices* can be blended into a salad dressing by adding a touch of vinegar, oil, and chopped fresh herbs. Juices are naturally rich in nutrients and enzymes and are low in fat.

Vegetable Broths, especially homemade broths, give body and flavor to soups, sauces, and one-pot grain dishes. Vegetable broths should replace commercial beef or chicken broths and bouillon cubes—many brands are high in fat and sodium.

White Wine can add a mellow nuance to soups, red sauces, sautéed vegetables, and risotto. White wine can replace most of the oil in sautéed dishes. For best results use dry wines such as Chardonnay or dry Riesling. Sweet wines (such as Zinfandel) can be used in fruity dishes.

Wine Mustard, also called Dijon-style mustard, has a sharp, pungent taste. The gourmet paste can thicken salad dressings, lowfat dairy sauces, and hearty soups such as mushroom and barley. Use mustard in place of mayonnaise as a sandwich spread.

Lowfat Dairy Products

Generally speaking, consumption of full-fat dairy products should be limited. However, there are healthful alternatives to whole milk, sour cream, and heavy cream.

A Cook's Guide to Lowfat Dairy Products

The healthy dairy products listed here are available in almost any supermarket.

Buttermilk is really low in fat (despite the name). Buttermilk makes a healthful alternative to milk, cream, and mayonnaise in creamy dressings, mashed potatoes, baked goods, and dips. Corn-bread and pumpkin muffins are especially good when made with buttermilk.

Lowfat Cottage Cheese, when puréed and combined with herbs and spices, makes a creamy lowfat dressing.

Lowfat Milk, with a little creativity, can replace full-fat heavy cream or whole milk in most sauces and soups. (Cornstarch or potatoes can thicken soups and sauces made with lowfat milk.) To give skim milk a richer flavor, combine equal parts of skim milk and soy milk.

Lowfat or *Nonfat Yogurt* makes an excellent substitute for sour cream in most recipes. Yogurt can also replace or extend mayonnaise and soft cheeses in many recipes. *Raita,* a classic sauce of chopped cucumbers and yogurt, is an excellent example of a lowfat yogurt sauce.

Field of Greens: Heart-Healthy Leafy Greens

Salads have long been the foundation of the health-minded lowfat diet. However, in many ways the typical American salad has been a grand deception. For starters, iceberg lettuce is the most bland and least nutritious of all the salad greens—yet it is the most popular lettuce offered in salad bars, in sandwiches, and on supermarket shelves. When iceberg lettuce is drenched with a creamy, high-fat dressing, the notion of a healthful meal falls apart.

On the other hand, there is a bounty of dark, nutritious leafy greens available at the marketplace. From the familiar red and green leaf, Romaine, and curly endive to willowy mizuna, red oak leaf, purple radicchio, and exotic greens in chartreuse, purple, and ruby maroon, there is a wide selection of salad greens far more enticing than iceberg lettuce. In general, the darker the leaf, the more nutritious the salad.

Dark leafy greens are high in carotenoids, vitamins A and C, folic acid, potassium, fiber, and other vitamins and minerals. Garnish the colorful leaves with an entourage of bright vegetables, and a healthful tossed salad is born.

Salad Preparation Tips

Selection: When shopping for leafy greens, inspect the leaves carefully. Choose greens that are crisp-looking and free of torn or discolored greens. When possible, shop for greens close to the date you are going to use them.

Preparation: Discard any damaged leaves. Remove the core with a twist of your hand or slice it with a knife; discard and trim off any fibrous stems.

Cleaning: Rinse the greens thoroughly. There is often sand and grit hiding between the leaves. Place the greens in a colander and rinse under cold running water, gently turning the greens. Or, place the greens in a colander set in a large bowl of cold water; gently swish the greens around, allowing the sand and grit to fall to the bottom. Let the greens sit for a few minutes and then drain.

Serving or Storing: Pat the leaves dry with a paper towel (or air-dry in a salad spinner). Toss the greens into a salad bowl or chill for later. To give chilled greens a crisp texture, wrap them in a paper towel and place in a perforated plastic bag. The greens are best when used within a few hours but will last for two or three days in the refrigerator.

Wait to Dress the Salad: Add the salad dressing at the last possible minute. Dressings cling to dry leaves but tend to slide off wet leaves and form a puddle at the bottom of the bowl.

Use a Mix of Greens: For optimal flavor and nutrients, mix and match a variety of greens. Pair a mild lettuce with an assertive green, flat leaves with curly leaves, green lettuces with red leaves.

A Cook's Guide to Salad Greens
The following is a guide to the many salad greens commonly found in well-stocked grocery stores and farmers' markets.

Arugula leaves are narrow, pale green, and oaklike in shape. Arugula has a spicy, peppery nuance and is ideally tossed with mild greens. The larger the leaf, the spicier the flavor.

Butterhead Lettuces, which include Bibb and Boston varieties, have a loose head with soft, ruffled leaves and a sweet flavor. Blend butterhead lettuce with an assertive green such as curly endive or frisee.

Curly Endive, also called chicory, has loose, frilly edges and a slightly bitter taste. Blend curly endive into salads with mild greens such as buttercrunch or oak leaf. Clean this green well (it tends to be sandy).

Frisee is a member of the chicory family. The narrow, pale green leaves have a jagged shape and feathery texture and a faint bitter taste. Frisee is popular in French cuisine.

Green Leaf is a loose head lettuce with wide ruffled leaves. This is the most versatile and widely available lettuce. Green leaf lettuce makes an excellent foundation for a tossed salad.

Mâche is a tender, mildly flavored green found at farmers' markets. It is best blended with a variety of other greens. Mâche is also called corn salad, field salad, and lamb's leaf.

Mesclun, the French term for "mixed field greens," is a blend of gourmet greens such as radicchio, oak leaf, frisee, mizuna, mâche, arugula, and chicory. Young, tender leaves (which do not require chopping) make the best mesclun salad.

Mizuna is a tender, narrow, Japanese leaf with ragged edges and mild mustardy flavor. Blend mizuna into a tossed salad of red and green leaf or buttercrunch lettuce.

Oak Leaf is a tender leaf lettuce with succulent flavor. (The leaves are shaped like large oak leaves.) It has a limited availability and is a popular offering at farmers' markets. Another enticing variety, red oak leaf, has a fringe of burgundy.

Radicchio is a small, tightly furled head with brilliant purplish red leaves streaked with white. Radicchio is also quite bitter and should be cut into thin strips and tossed with other leafy greens.

Red Leaf, also called ruby lettuce, is the cousin of green leaf. The loose, furled leaves are marked with a reddish maroon trim. For a colorful salad, combine red leaf with green leaf and oak leaf.

Romaine Lettuce has crisp, oblong leaves that vary from dark green to light green. Romaine is used in Caesar salads and gourmet sandwiches. To prepare Romaine lettuce, cut the broad leaves into ribbonlike strips and combine with other greens.

Spinach makes a nutritious addition to any tossed salad. The dark green leaves are high in beta-carotene, vitamin C, fiber, iron, and other nutrients.

Watercress is a spry herb that doubles as a salad garnish. The small oval leaves come attached to long stems. The flavor of watercress ranges from mild to spicy.

Salad Wish List
Every time you add a garnish to the salad bowl you not only enhance the flavors—you also contribute many essential phytonutrients. See Tables 3.3 and 3.4.

TABLE 3.3
Healthy Salad Garnishes

Salad Garnish	Health Benefits
Tomato wedges	Lycopene and vitamin C
Shredded carrots	Carotenoids and fiber
Shredded red cabbage	A phytochemical powerhouse
Slivered red onion	Over fifty phytochemicals, including sulfides and quercetin
Shredded beet roots	Raw beets are a natural diuretic
Red kidney beans or chick-peas	Fiber and protein
Red bell pepper rings	Vitamin C and beta-carotene
Hot chili peppers	Capsaicin (a phytochemical)
Broccoli and cauliflower florets	Vitamin A, carotenoids, and phytochemicals (sulforaphane and indoles)
Dried fruit such as raisins, apricots, and dates	Iron, potassium, and fiber
Raspberries, blueberries, and strawberries	Vitamin C and ellagic acid (a phytochemical)
Nuts and seeds (unsalted pumpkin seeds, sunflower seeds, walnuts, or cashews)	Fiber, protein, vitamin E, and unsaturated fats
Diced nectarines, peaches, mangos, pineapple, and star fruit	Fiber, vitamin C, and carotenoids

TABLE 3.4
Salad Do's and Don'ts

Do's	Don'ts
Do include a variety of dark leafy greens in the salad bowl.	Don't buy iceberg lettuce.
Do choose a vinaigrette, fruit purée, or balsamic vinegar as a dressing.	Don't cover your salad with creamy, full-fat dressings (such as Thousand Island, creamy bleu cheese, or Russian).
Do include a variety of raw vegetables in your salad bowl.	Don't add luncheon meats, bacon, or boiled egg yolks.
Do include exotic garnishes such as jicama, sprouts, radicchio, arugula, and roasted tofu.	Don't go overboard with shredded cheeses or crumbled cheese such as bleu cheese, Roquefort, or feta.
Do include a variety of legumes, nuts, and seeds.	Don't include high-sodium ingredients such as imitation bacon bits, crackers, or commercial croutons.

SIGNATURE RECIPES FOR THE LOWFAT, LOW-CHOLESTEROL, HEALTHY DIET

Classic Salad Vinaigrette

Kiwi Vinaigrette

Tropical Fruit Chutney

Cucumber Yogurt Sauce

Black Bean and Tomato Salsa

Vegetable Topping for Soup and Chili

Sweet Potato Bisque

Lime-Basted Sweet Corn

Lemon-Dill Asparagus Spears

Black Bean and Brown Rice Jambalaya

Creole Vegetable Hot Pot

Vegetable Couscous

Perfect Marinara Sauce

Pasta with Oven-Broiled Vegetables

Pasta with Mushroom-Tarragon Primavera

Macaroni Ratatouille

Penne Pasta with Lemony Swiss Chard

Very Berry Cornbread

Orange-Zucchini Muffins

Apple-Raspberry Muffins

Additional health benefits are noted with each recipe.

Classic Salad Vinaigrette

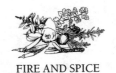

FIRE AND SPICE

This vinaigrette is a versatile dressing for tossed salads and can also replace the mayonnaise in pasta or potato salads. It can also be drizzled over steamed or roasted vegetables in place of butter.

- ¼ cup canola oil (plus 2 tablespoons, optional)
- 3 tablespoons red wine vinegar
- 1 tablespoon balsamic vinegar or rice vinegar
- 1½ teaspoons Dijon-style mustard
- 2 teaspoons honey
- 2 teaspoons *mixture* of dried herbs (oregano, basil, parsley, and thyme)
- ½ teaspoon black pepper
- ¼ teaspoon salt
- 2 tablespoons chopped fresh herbs (basil, parsley, or mint)

Combine all of the ingredients in a mixing bowl and whisk thoroughly. Refrigerate for 30 minutes to allow the flavors to meld together.

Serve as a dressing for almost any green salad or toss the dressing with a pasta or rice salad.

YIELD: ABOUT ⅔ CUP (4 TO 6 SERVINGS)

HELPFUL HINT

Make extra vinaigrette and store the leftover dressing in the refrigerator. The vinaigrette mellows as the flavors mingle together. If kept refrigerated, a vinaigrette will keep for several weeks. Whisk or shake well before serving.

Kiwi Vinaigrette

ANTIOXIDANTS

FIRE AND SPICE

Puréed kiwi fruits form the basis of this creamy dressing. In addition to inspiring this lowfat dressing, kiwi fruits are also loaded with vitamin C.

4 kiwi fruits, peeled and coarsely chopped
$1/4$ cup red wine vinegar or apple cider vinegar
$1/4$ cup canola oil
1 tablespoon honey
$1/2$ teaspoon white pepper
$1/4$ teaspoon salt

Place all of the ingredients in a blender or food processor fitted with a steel blade. Process for about 10 seconds until smooth and creamy. Pour into a serving container and serve at once or refrigerate for later.

YIELD: ABOUT 2 CUPS (12 SERVINGS)

HELPFUL HINT

Use ripe, sweet kiwi fruits. You can determine the ripeness by holding the kiwi in the palm of your hand and gently pressing down with your thumb; it should give a little.

Tropical Fruit Chutney

This sweet-and-tart condiment is overflowing with tropical fruits and deep aromatic flavors. Serve the chutney over baked potatoes, grilled fish, or steamed green vegetables or as a substitute for butter on scones and biscuits.

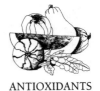

ANTIOXIDANTS

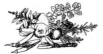

FIRE AND SPICE

1 cup diced fresh pineapple
1 mango, peeled, pitted, and diced
1 papaya, peeled, seeded, and diced
1 medium red onion, diced
2 to 3 cloves garlic, minced
1 tablespoon minced fresh ginger
³/4 cup red wine vinegar
¹/2 cup apple cider
¹/3 cup brown sugar
¹/2 teaspoon ground cloves
¹/2 teaspoon ground cumin
¹/2 teaspoon black pepper
¹/4 teaspoon salt

Place all of the ingredients in a nonreactive saucepan. Cook over medium heat for about 15 to 20 minutes, stirring occasionally. Lower the heat as the mixture begins to thicken.

Allow the chutney to cool to room temperature, then refrigerate. If refrigerated, the chutney should keep for several weeks.

YIELD: ABOUT 2¹/2 CUPS

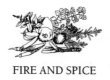

Cucumber Yogurt Sauce

This soothing condiment can be served with chili, curry dishes, stews, and bean soups. It also can replace the sour cream topping used for baked potatoes.

2 cups plain lowfat yogurt
1 cup finely chopped cucumbers
2 tablespoons chopped fresh mint or parsley
   (or 1 tablespoon dried)

Combine all of the ingredients in a mixing bowl. Cover and chill until ready to serve.

YIELD: 3 CUPS (ABOUT 6 TO 8 SERVINGS)

Black Bean and Tomato Salsa

While there are many varieties of salsa, the core flavors are cilantro, lime, and chili peppers (most often jalapeños). This tangy trio of flavors produces the essence of salsa.

2 ripe tomatoes, diced
1 red bell pepper, seeded and diced
1 medium yellow onion, diced
2 large cloves garlic, minced
1 jalapeño pepper, seeded and minced
2 tablespoons chopped fresh cilantro
Juice of 1 lime
1 teaspoon ground cumin
1 teaspoon dried oregano
$^1/_2$ teaspoon black pepper
$^1/_4$ teaspoon salt
1 can (16 ounces) crushed tomatoes
1 cup canned black beans, drained

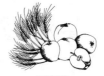

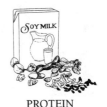

Combine all of the ingredients except the crushed tomatoes and beans in a large bowl and mix well. Place three-quarters of the mixture in a food processor fitted with a steel blade and process for 5 seconds, creating a chunky vegetable mash.

Return the mash to the bowl and add the crushed tomatoes and beans; blend well. Chill the salsa for at least 1 hour to allow the flavors to meld together. Serve with warm flour tortillas.

YIELD: 4$^1/_2$ CUPS

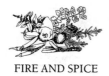

Vegetable Topping for Soup and Chili

This easy-to-prepare mixture of crunchy vegetables and nuts makes a perfect complementary garnish to well-cooked soups, chili, stews, and soy-based stir-fries. Skip the sour cream and reach for the veggies!

4 whole scallions, sliced diagonally
2 ounces mung bean sprouts
1 red radish, chopped
2 tablespoons chopped cashews (unsalted)

Combine all of the ingredients in a medium mixing bowl. Transfer to a serving dish. At the last minute, sprinkle the mixture over bean soups, chili, tomato-based soups, stir-fries, pilafs, and root vegetable stews.

YIELD: ABOUT 4 SERVINGS

Sweet Potato Bisque

Here is delicious proof that not every bisque must drip with heavy cream and butter.

1 tablespoon canola oil
1 medium yellow onion, diced
1 red bell pepper, seeded and diced
2 stalks celery, chopped
2 large cloves garlic, minced
4 cups coarsely chopped sweet potatoes (peeled if desired)
2 teaspoons paprika
1½ teaspoons ground cumin
½ teaspoon salt
½ teaspoon white pepper
1 cup dairy milk or soy milk
2 tablespoons chopped fresh cilantro (optional)

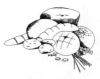

In a large saucepan heat the oil over medium heat. Add the onion, bell pepper, celery, and garlic and cook, stirring, for about 5 minutes. Add 4 cups water, the sweet potatoes, paprika, cumin, salt, and pepper and bring to a simmer. Cook over medium-low heat until the potatoes are tender, about 20 minutes, stirring occasionally.

Transfer the soup to a blender or food processor fitted with a steel blade and purée until smooth, about 5 seconds. Return the soup to the pan and stir in the milk. Bring the soup to a gentle simmer.

Ladle the bisque into bowls and sprinkle with cilantro. Serve at once.

YIELD: 6 SERVINGS

Lime-Basted Sweet Corn

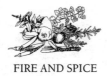

It is no secret that fresh corn tastes best when it is picked, cooked, and eaten within hours. Fresh corn doesn't require a lot of embellishment and certainly does not need butter. A touch of lime and cayenne pepper will suffice.

    4 to 6 ears of corn, shucked
    2 limes, quartered
    Cayenne pepper, to taste

Place the corn in a large pot of boiling water. Cook the corn for 3 to 7 minutes over medium-high heat, stirring occasionally. Drain in a colander.

Rub the wedges of lime over the corn and sprinkle with cayenne pepper. Eat at once.

YIELD: 4 SERVINGS

Lemon-Dill Asparagus Spears

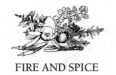

FIRE AND SPICE

Asparagus are a truly regal vegetable, but unfortunately they are often drowned in hollandaise sauce or butter sauces. This blend of lemon and herbs enhances the asparagus spears without flooding them in a pool of fat.

Juice of 1$^{1}/_{2}$ lemons
2 tablespoons olive oil
1 tablespoon chopped fresh dill
$^{1}/_{2}$ teaspoon white pepper
$^{1}/_{2}$ teaspoon salt
$^{1}/_{2}$ cup roasted sweet peppers, chopped
1 pound asparagus spears, fibrous ends removed
2 tablespoons chopped fresh parsley

In a small mixing bowl whisk together the lemon juice, olive oil, dill, pepper, and salt. Stir in the roasted sweet peppers and set aside.

Bring about 1 quart of water to a boil in a medium saucepan. Place the asparagus in the boiling water and cook over medium heat until tender, 3 to 4 minutes. Drain in a colander. (Alternatively, you may steam the asparagus until tender.)

In a large mixing bowl, gently toss the asparagus with the lemon dressing. Arrange the spears on an oval platter and top with the parsley. Serve warm as a side dish.

YIELD: 4 SERVINGS

Black Bean and Brown Rice Jambalaya

ANTIOXIDANTS

FIBER

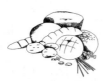

PROTEIN

POWER EATING

Here is vivid proof that a great jambalaya need not include sausages, poultry, or fatty meats. This healthy adaptation is hearty, robust, and filled with good-for-you nutrients.

1½ cups brown rice
1 tablespoon canola oil
12 button mushrooms, sliced
1 green bell pepper, seeded and diced
1 medium yellow onion, diced
1 large celery stalk, diced
3 or 4 cloves garlic, minced
1 can (15 ounces) tomato purée
1 can (14 ounces) stewed tomatoes
1 can (15 ounces) black beans, drained
1 tablespoon dried oregano
½ teaspoon black pepper
¼ teaspoon cayenne pepper
1 to 2 teaspoons bottled hot sauce (such as Tabasco)

In a medium saucepan combine the rice and 3¼ cups water and bring to a simmer over medium-high heat. Stir the rice, turn the heat down to medium-low, and cover the pan; cook for 30 minutes until all of the liquid is absorbed. Remove from the heat and let stand for 5 to 10 minutes.

In a large saucepan heat the oil over medium heat. Add the mushrooms, bell pepper, onion, celery, and garlic and cook, stirring, for 7 to 8 minutes. Add the tomato purée, stewed tomatoes, beans, oregano, pepper, cayenne, and hot sauce and cook over medium-low heat for 15 minutes, stirring occasionally. Fold in the cooked rice and cook for 4 minutes more over low heat.

Ladle the jambalaya into shallow bowls and serve with braised greens.

YIELD: 6 SERVINGS

HELPFUL HINT

If you want to include seafood in this dish, add about $3/4$ pound of medium shrimp (peeled) or sea scallops to the pan after you've added the vegetables. Cook for a few minutes and continue with the recipe.

Creole Vegetable Hot Pot

ANTIOXIDANTS

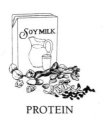

FIBER

PROTEIN

A traditional Creole sauce includes onion, peppers, celery, tomatoes, and plenty of spices—and is naturally low in fat. This meatless Creole dish is stocked with sturdy vegetables.

1 tablespoon canola oil
2 cups diced eggplant
1 medium yellow onion, diced
1 green bell pepper, seeded and diced
1 large celery stalk, chopped
3 or 4 cloves garlic, minced
1 can (28 ounces) stewed tomatoes
1 can (15 ounces) red kidney beans, drained
1 tablespoon dried oregano
1 teaspoon dried thyme
1/2 teaspoon black pepper
1/4 teaspoon cayenne pepper
1/2 teaspoon salt
1 to 2 teaspoons of your favorite bottled hot sauce

In a large saucepan heat the oil over medium heat. Add the eggplant, onion, bell pepper, celery, and garlic. Cook, stirring, until the vegetables are tender, about 8 minutes. Add the stewed tomatoes, beans, oregano, thyme, black pepper, cayenne, and salt and cook over medium-low heat for 15 to 20 minutes, stirring occasionally. Stir in the hot sauce and let stand for 5 to 10 minutes before serving.

Serve the Creole vegetables over brown rice or pasta.

YIELD: 6 SERVINGS

Vegetable Couscous

This lightly flavored dish of vegetables and fluffy couscous makes a light dinner or substantial side dish.

ANTIOXIDANTS

1   tablespoon canola oil
1   medium yellow onion, diced
1   red bell pepper, seeded and diced
2   large cloves garlic, minced
3   cups coarsely chopped chard or spinach
2   teaspoons dried oregano
1/2 teaspoon salt
1/2 teaspoon black pepper
2   cups whole wheat couscous
1   can (15 ounces) chick-peas, drained
4   whole scallions, chopped
Juice of 1 large lemon or lime

PROTEIN

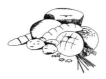

POWER EATING

In a large saucepan heat the oil over medium high heat. Add the onion, bell pepper, and garlic and cook, stirring, for about 5 minutes. Add 3 cups water, the greens, oregano, salt, and pepper and bring to a simmer. Cook, stirring, for 3 to 4 minutes. Stir in the couscous, chick-peas, and scallions, cover the pan, and turn off the heat. Let stand for 10 minutes.

Fluff the couscous and fold in the citrus juice. Serve at once.

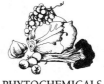

PHYTOCHEMICALS

YIELD: 4 SERVINGS

Perfect Marinara Sauce

ANTIOXIDANTS

Aficionados of Italian food know that canned plum tomatoes make the best homemade marinara sauce. Plum tomatoes have a thick flesh and robust flavor.

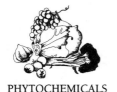

PHYTOCHEMICALS

1   tablespoon olive oil
1   medium yellow onion, diced
2   large cloves garlic, minced
1   can (28 ounces) plum tomatoes
1/4 cup chopped fresh parsley
1   teaspoon sugar (optional)
1 1/2 teaspoons dried oregano
1   teaspoon dried basil
1/2 teaspoon black pepper
1/2 teaspoon salt
1/2 cup chopped fresh basil (optional)

In a large saucepan heat the oil over medium heat. Add the onion and garlic and cook, stirring, for 4 minutes. Add the plum tomatoes, parsley, sugar, oregano, basil, pepper, and salt and bring to a simmer. Cook for 20 minutes over low heat, stirring occasionally.

Transfer the sauce to a food processor fitted with a steel blade or to a blender and process for about 5 seconds until smooth. Return the sauce to the pan and keep warm until the pasta is ready. Stir in the fresh basil before serving.

YIELD: 4 SERVINGS

Pasta with Oven-Broiled Vegetables

Pasta goes with just about every vegetable on the planet. For this dish linguini is tossed with a medley of broiled and lightly dressed vegetables.

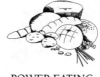

POWER EATING

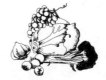

PHYTOCHEMICALS

1   tablespoon olive oil
2   tablespoons red wine vinegar
2   tablespoons chopped fresh parsley
1   teaspoon dried oregano
$^1/_4$ teaspoon cayenne pepper
$^1/_2$ teaspoon salt
1   zucchini, quartered lengthwise
1   medium red onion, quartered
1   red bell pepper, cored
3   or 4 portobello mushrooms
8   ounces linguini or spaghetti

In a large mixing bowl combine the olive oil, vinegar, parsley, oregano, cayenne, and salt. Set aside.

Preheat the oven broiler.

Arrange the vegetables on a baking sheet. Place beneath the broiler and broil for about 5 minutes on each side until the vegetables are tender. Remove the vegetables as they become done and transfer to a cutting board; let cool slightly and coarsely chop. Toss the vegetables with the dressing.

Meanwhile, in a large saucepan bring 3 quarts of water to a boil over medium-high heat. Place the pasta in the boiling water, stir, and return to a boil. Cook for 8 to 10 minutes until al dente, stirring occasionally. Drain in a colander.

Add the pasta to the roasted vegetables and toss together. Serve at once.

YIELD: 4 SERVINGS

Pasta with Mushroom-Tarragon Primavera

This lighter version of primavera exudes the earthy flavors of wild mushrooms and tarragon.

8 ounces linguini or spaghetti
1 tablespoon canola oil
1 tablespoon dry white wine
8 ounces button mushrooms, sliced
6 to 8 fresh shiitake mushrooms, sliced
4 ounces oyster mushrooms, sliced
4 cloves garlic, minced
2 cups lowfat milk
2 tablespoons chopped fresh parsley
1¹/₂ tablespoons Dijon-style mustard
1 teaspoon dried tarragon
¹/₂ teaspoon white pepper
¹/₂ teaspoon salt
2 tablespoons cornstarch
2 tablespoons cold water

In a large saucepan bring 3 quarts of water to a boil over medium-high heat. Place the linguini in the boiling water, stir, and return to a boil. Cook until al dente, about 8 to 10 minutes, stirring occasionally. Drain the linguini in a colander.

In another large saucepan heat the oil and wine over medium-high heat. Add the mushrooms and garlic and cook, stirring, for 6 to 8 minutes. Stir in the milk, parsley, mustard, tarragon, pepper, and salt and bring to a gentle simmer over medium heat.

Meanwhile, in a small mixing bowl combine the cornstarch and water. Stir the slurry mixture into the simmering sauce and return to a gentle simmer. Fold in the cooked linguini. Cook for about 1 minute more over low heat, stirring frequently.

Transfer the noodles to warm serving plates and serve at once.

YIELD: 4 SERVINGS

VARIATION

For a low-sodium version, add the juice of 1 lemon a few minutes before serving and omit the salt.

Macaroni Ratatouille

ANTIOXIDANTS

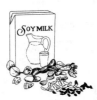

FIBER

PROTEIN

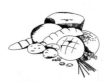

POWER EATING

This satisfying one-pot meal is a take-off on the classic Mediterranean dish. For variety, try elbow macaroni made with spelt, quinoa, or corn.

1   cup elbow macaroni
2   tablespoons dry red wine
1   tablespoon canola oil
1   medium yellow onion, diced
1   green bell pepper, seeded and diced
8   ounces button mushrooms, sliced
2   cups diced eggplant
3   or 4 cloves garlic, minced
1   can (28 ounces) plum or stewed tomatoes
1   can (15 ounces) red kidney beans, drained
2   teaspoons dried oregano
1   teaspoon dried basil
1/2 teaspoon black pepper
1/2 teaspoon salt

In a large saucepan bring 3 quarts of water to a boil over medium-high heat. Place the macaroni in the boiling water, stir, and return to a boil. Cook until al dente, about 6 minutes, stirring occasionally. Drain in a colander.

Meanwhile, in another large saucepan heat the wine and oil over medium heat. Add the onion, bell pepper, mushrooms, eggplant, and garlic and cook, stirring, for about 10 minutes over medium heat until the vegetables are tender. Stir in the canned plum or stewed tomatoes, beans, oregano, basil, pepper, and salt and bring to a simmer. Cook over medium-low heat for 15 minutes, stirring occasionally. (Cut the tomatoes into smaller pieces with the edge of a large spoon.)

Remove from the heat and fold in the macaroni. Ladle the ratatouille into shallow bowls and serve with warm Italian bread.

YIELD: 6 SERVINGS

Penne Pasta with Lemony Swiss Chard

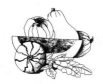

ANTIOXIDANTS

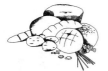

POWER EATING

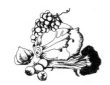

PHYTOCHEMICALS

This side dish of pasta and braised greens is flavored with a hint of lemon and garlic. You won't miss the cream, eggs, or cheese.

1 bunch red or green chard leaves
2 teaspoons olive oil or canola oil
1 medium yellow onion, chopped
2 or 3 cloves garlic, minced
$^1/_2$ teaspoon salt
$^1/_2$ teaspoon black pepper
Juice of 1 large lemon
8 ounces penne or ziti pasta

Remove the fibrous stems of the chard leaves and discard. Rinse the leaves and cut into ribbons (chiffonade-style).

In a large, wide skillet heat the oil over medium heat. Add the onion and garlic and cook, stirring, for 3 minutes. Stir in the chard, salt, pepper, and lemon juice. Cook for about 5 minutes, stirring frequently, until the greens are wilted and tender. Set aside.

Meanwhile, in a large saucepan bring $2^1/_2$ quarts of water to a boil over medium-high heat. Place the pasta in the boiling water, stir, and return to a boil. Cook until al dente, about 8 to 10 minutes, stirring occasionally. Drain in a colander.

Add the pasta to the braised greens and toss together. Serve at once.

YIELD: 4 SERVINGS

Very Berry Cornbread

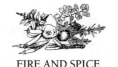

Adding fruit to breads and desserts is an easy way to "up" the nutrient content (and flavor) and reduce the fat.

1   cup yellow cornmeal
1   cup unbleached all-purpose flour
$^1/_3$ cup sugar
1   tablespoon baking powder
$^1/_2$ teaspoon salt
1   egg, beaten, plus 1 egg white
1   cup dairy milk or soy milk
3   tablespoons canola oil
$1^1/_2$ cups blueberries, fresh or frozen and thawed

Preheat the oven to 375 degrees F.

Combine the cornmeal, flour, sugar, baking powder, and salt in a mixing bowl. In a separate bowl, whisk together the eggs, milk or soy milk, and oil. Gently fold the liquid ingredients into the dry ingredients until a batter is formed. Fold in the blueberries.

Pour the batter into a lightly greased 8-inch square baking pan. Bake for 20 to 25 minutes, until the crust is almost light brown and a toothpick inserted in the center comes out clean. Remove from the heat and let cool for a few minutes before cutting.

YIELD: 8 TO 10 SERVINGS

Orange-Zucchini Muffins

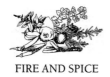

FIRE AND SPICE

These moist muffins have significantly less fat than normal muffins—but double the flavor! Orange juice replaces half the oil, and butter is completely out of the picture.

$^1/_2$ cup orange juice
$^1/_2$ cup canola oil
1 cup brown sugar
1 large egg and 1 egg white, beaten
1 tablespoon orange zest
2 cups unbleached all-purpose flour
1 tablespoon baking powder
1 teaspoon salt
1 teaspoon ground cinnamon
1 teaspoon ground nutmeg
2 cups grated zucchini
$^1/_2$ cup raisins or 1 cup diced walnuts (or both)
$^1/_4$ cup rolled oatmeal

Preheat the oven to 350 degrees F.

In a large mixing bowl combine the juice, oil, sugar, eggs, and orange zest; whisk until the batter is creamy. In a separate bowl combine the flour, baking powder, salt, cinnamon, and nutmeg. Fold into the liquid ingredients, forming a batter. Gently fold in the zucchini and raisins and/or walnuts.

Pour the batter into a lightly greased muffin tin. Sprinkle a little oatmeal over each muffin. Place in the oven and bake for 20 to 25 minutes, until a toothpick inserted in the center comes out clean. Remove from the heat and let cool for about 10 minutes before serving.

YIELD: 10 TO 12 MUFFINS

Apple-Raspberry Muffins

These fruity muffins contain half the fat, twice the nutrients, and triple the flavor of traditional muffins.

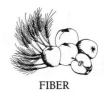

FIBER

$1/2$ cup orange juice
$1/2$ cup canola oil
1 cup granulated sugar
1 cup brown sugar
1 large egg and 1 large egg white
4 cups diced apples
$1^1/2$ cups fresh raspberries
2 cups unbleached all-purpose flour
1 cup whole wheat flour
1 tablespoon baking powder
1 teaspoon salt
1 teaspoon ground nutmeg
1 teaspoon ground cinnamon
1 cup diced walnuts or pecans
$1/4$ cup oatmeal

Preheat the oven to 375 degrees F.

In a large mixing bowl blend together the orange juice, oil, and sugars until fully incorporated. Beat in the eggs. Fold in the apples and raspberries.

In a separate medium mixing bowl combine the flour, baking powder, salt, nutmeg, and cinnamon. Fold the dry mixture into the wet batter. Fold in the nuts.

Pour the batter into muffin tins (sprayed with vegetable oil). Place the pans on the middle rack in the oven and bake for 50 to 55 minutes until a toothpick inserted in the center comes out clean. Set on a rack to cool for 30 minutes.

YIELD: 12 MUFFINS

Pillar 4

EXPLODING THE PROTEIN MYTHS

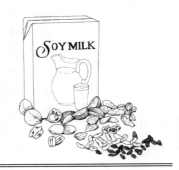

W HEN THE SUPPER HOUR ARRIVES IN AMERICA, ANI-
mal foods dominate the menu. Red meat, poultry, and seafood fill
the center of the plate while nutritious plant foods—vegetables,
grains, potatoes, beans, and rice—are relegated to small portions
on the side. As with its penchant for baseball and apple pie, this
country has a tremendous appetite for hot dogs, hamburgers, pork
chops, and roasted chicken. The nation is hooked on meat.

Our national dependency on animal food is graphically demonstrated at the supermarket checkout line. Caravans of grocery
carts line up with massive cargoes of shrink-wrapped meat products destined for the dinner table. From tenderloin, sirloin tip,
filet mignon, pork chops, and leg of lamb to brisket, top round,
London broil, and ground beef (and ground chuck), the array of
red meat is astounding. The poultry and sausage sections are just
as expansive, as is the processed meats department filled with
slick packages of bacon, cured meats, cold cuts, and turkey
sausages. In their variety and merchandising space, the sprawling
meat departments rank a close second to the canyonesque junk
foods aisle.

The nation's booming restaurant scene also highlights dishes laden with beef, pork, poultry, and fish. When vegetarian entrées are offered, the choices are usually limited and uncreative—oftentimes it's a tossed salad or quiche. The resources of the kitchen are devoted to meaty foods, not developing meatless entrées (ironically, meatless meals are also more profitable). In all fairness, the restaurant industry is simply meeting the demands of a carnivorous public with a huge appetite for meat, chicken, and fish.

A PENCHANT FOR PROTEIN

How did we become such a meat-devouring, chicken-nibbling, burger-chowing culture? There are many reasons. For starters, meat is available to the masses, affordable, and conveniently packaged. Meat is ready to go and easy to prepare—important factors in our time-challenged society. Animal foods are also perceived by many as the best food source for protein, iron, and zinc (all debatable points). Habits and routine play a large role—most of us grew up with meat on the table. Holiday and family gatherings revolve around roast turkey and baked ham. (I'm sure most people think a vegetarian Thanksgiving is an oxymoron.)

The zeal for meat can also be attributed to the mores of the times. For decades nutritionists have preached about the virtues of protein and amino acids, the building blocks for proper growth and development. Millions of Americans got the message, and today the typical American diet is saddled with an excess of animal protein. In fact, it has been estimated that the average American diet contains twice as much protein as the recommended daily allowance. Much of this surplus is eliminated as waste, not stored as muscle. (It has been observed that Americans have the most expensive urine in the world.) The push for protein also parallels the alarming increase of dietary fat and cholesterol.

Across the board, the average diet consumes a fraction of the recommended fiber, a pittance of antioxidants and phytonutrients, way too much fat, and double the amount of required protein. Unfortunately, the popular penchant for protein is not without serious repercussions. The nation's love affair with animal food and protein comes with a hefty price tag.

THE TROUBLE(S) WITH ANIMAL PROTEIN

Animal proteins travel with artery-clogging saturated fat and cholesterol, two significant risk factors for heart disease, obesity, stroke, hypertension, and other ailments. Even in the absence of saturated fat and cholesterol, animal protein has been linked with elevated cholesterol levels. On the other hand, plant proteins come with little fat and contain no cholesterol. (For more on the animal protein–cholesterol connection, turn to Pillar 3: Treasures of the Heart: Secrets of Lowfat, Low-Cholesterol Cooking.)

Diets with excessive animal protein can be linked to cancer. There is emerging evidence linking excessive meat and dairy consumption (i.e., animal proteins) with prostate cancer and colon cancer. Also, in populations where animal protein consumption is low, the colon and prostate cancer rates are low. (Critics argue that people who eat excessive amounts of animal protein also tend to consume plenty of saturated fat and less fiber and antioxidants, other risk factors contributing to chronic disease. Therefore, some say, because fat and animal protein are often consumed together, it is hard to prove the protein link with cancer.)

Dr. Colin Campbell, a professor of nutritional biochemistry at Cornell University, blames the typical high-protein, animal-based diet for a range of health problems, including coronary heart disease, osteoporosis, and certain cancers. According to Dr. Campbell, when animal proteins are exposed to carcinogens in animal studies, the tumors grow and multiply as if fed by the animal protein. When tumors are exposed to plant-based soy proteins, the growth slows or reverses. Dating back over fifty years, there have been numerous studies that support the contention that animals

The nation's love affair with animal food and protein comes with a hefty price tag.

Animal proteins travel with artery-clogging saturated fat and cholesterol.

fed high-protein diets will develop more tumors than those fed low-protein or plant-protein diets.

Protein-rich animal foods are conspicuously lacking in many of the disease-fighting substances found in plant foods. Beef and chicken dishes are deficient in fiber, antioxidants, phytochemicals, and energy-supplying complex carbohydrates. Furthermore, if a plate is loaded with a porterhouse steak or barbecued ribs, there is little room in the appetite for other, more healthful foods with protective micronutrients (of course, there always seems to be room for dessert!).

The human ability to digest animal foods is being scrutinized. Beef, chicken, and pork are concentrated sources of protein, a nutrient that consists of amino *acids*. Meat also contains plenty of saturated fat, which is made of fatty *acids*. Meat eaters often experience indigestion and gastric distress after a typical meal (and often feel lethargic as well). Put two and two together. No wonder the American population is addicted to *antacids*, a billion-dollar industry. Perhaps many episodes of indigestion are caused by the acid-rich meat and fat in the spaghetti sauce and chili, not by the spices. (Hot peppers may actually facilitate digestion by stimulating the release of digestive enzymes.)

Surprisingly, there are now over-the-counter pills designed to be swallowed before eating a dinner rich in meat and fat. (The question begs to be asked: If you know ahead of time that the dish is going to upset your stomach and wreak havoc with your intestines, why eat it in the first place? Inquiring minds want to know.) Meanwhile, commercials for heartburn relief and antacids are all over the television and radio airwaves, and kitchen cupboards fill up with economy-size containers of antacids. Go figure.

Aside from the compelling nutritional concerns, there are plenty of sociopolitical reasons to be wary of animal foods. Good and upstanding citizens will argue passionately over the political and environmental ramifications of raising and killing animals for food. (If you want to become a vegetarian overnight, arrange for a tour of a slaughterhouse.) Others point to the risk of food-related

Protein-rich animal foods are conspicuously lacking in many of the disease-fighting substances found in plant foods.

The human ability to digest animal foods is under scrutiny.

Aside from the compelling nutritional concerns, there are plenty of sociopolitical reasons to be wary of animal foods.

illnesses stemming from improperly prepared red meat, poultry, or seafood dishes. There have been several well-known outbreaks linked to tainted meats. The words *E. coli* and *salmonella* are familiar to the public.

Compared to a plant-based diet teeming with nutrient-rich vegetables, grains, legumes, and fruits, foods of animal origin make negligible contributions to your long-term health and well-being. Dr. Neal Barnard, president of Physicians Committee for Responsible Medicine, has compared the health hazards of eating meat over the course of a lifetime with the dangers of smoking tobacco—pretty strong stuff.

Sadly, despite the preponderance of detrimental characteristics associated with a protein-rich, meat-based diet, animal foods continue to dominate the American dinner table.

THE MULTIPLE MYTHS ABOUT MEAT AND PROTEIN

Myth #1: Without meat in our diet, we would suffer from protein deficiency.

The reality: A well-balanced diet of vegetables, fruits, grains, and legumes supplies an ample amount of protein to meet our body's needs.

Myth #2: Proteins derived from red meat, poultry, pork, fish, and dairy products offer "complete" proteins. Vegetable proteins are incomplete, and therefore inferior.

The reality: True, animal foods offer "complete" proteins because they contain all nine essential amino acids that our bodies need. However, when the "incomplete" vegetable proteins are combined in a meal, complementary amino acids team up to form complete proteins. This is not a rare event; there are hundreds of potential combinations of vegetables, grains, legumes, and fruits to choose from.

Myth #3: High-protein diets will help athletes build bigger muscles and increase overall strength and stamina.

The reality: Muscles get bigger from pumping iron, not from eating steaks or guzzling protein shakes. High-protein diets will not help athletes run faster or jump higher—practice and exercise will do that. Protein is also not the most optimal source of energy—complex carbohydrates more efficiently fill that role. If a high-performance athlete maintains a well-balanced diet with plenty of vegetables, grains, and beans, the protein needs will be met.

Myth #4: You can never eat too much protein.

The reality: To the contrary, experts believe that a lifetime of excessive consumption of animal protein can contribute to myriad health problems. High protein intake has been associated with calcium depletion (a precursor to osteoporosis and weak bones), kidney damage, and certain cancers. There is also evidence shedding light on animal protein's role in elevating blood cholesterol and thereby contributing to heart disease.

In the long run, too much animal protein in your diet can be detrimental to your health. For these reasons, the safety of fad-driven, high-protein diets must also be questioned.

Myth #5: Meat is the best source of iron and zinc. Avoiding animal protein would cause a deficiency of these essential minerals.

The reality: Well, not exactly. The "iron and zinc" defense is often employed but not entirely true. Soy foods (tofu, soy milk) contain both minerals. Beans, dark leafy greens, fruit, prunes, dried apricots, and raisins are all good sources of iron. Oatmeal, whole grain cereals and breads, and wheat germ are good sources of zinc.

Myth #6: Vegetarians can suffer from vitamin B-12 deficiencies.

The reality: It is true that vitamin B-12 is the one nutrient that is not in plentiful supply in plant foods. B-12 is produced by bacteria and is essential for maintaining healthy nerves. The actual daily need is quite small since the body stores B-12 (there is not a daily requirement). In addition, most cereals and breads are enriched with the vitamin. Miso and tempeh (soy food products) also contain B-12. There is speculation that organic vegetables may retain B-12 when grown in certain conditions. Stay tuned as more is learned about this essential nutrient.

PROTEIN'S ROLE IN A HEALTHY DIET: AN IN-DEPTH LOOK

To fully understand the role of protein in a healthy diet and to appreciate the intensity of the debate, it is important to wade through the hype and the headlines and explore the basic tenets of this essential nutrient.

Despite the abundance of popular myths, protein does play an important role in the healthy diet. The word *protein* is derived from a Greek term meaning "primary," or "of first importance." Protein performs many life-sustaining tasks such as replenishing muscles, forming enzymes and hormones, repairing and building tissue, and helping to fight off infections by producing antibodies. Protein is an indispensable component in our bones, organs, and body fluids. Without a doubt, all life depends on protein.

PROTEIN STARTS WITH AMINO ACIDS

To understand your body's protein needs, it is necessary to come to grips with amino acids, the building blocks of protein. Every complete protein consists of a chain of 22 amino acids, most of which have tongue-twisting names like tryptophan, lysine, leucine, and valine. Of these 22 amino acids required to assemble a complete protein, your body manufactures only 13. That means that the remaining 9 amino acids must be derived from your diet and are considered essential to your health.

Animal foods contain all 22 amino acids and offer "one-stop shopping" for your protein requirements. A meal prepared with either meat, poultry, seafood, eggs, or dairy products will provide the body with ready-to-use complete proteins. On the other hand, individual plant foods contain varying types of amino acids but do not offer all 9 essential amino acids at once. By themselves, plant-based foods such as vegetables, grains, legumes, and fruits offer "incomplete" proteins, since one or more amino acids are missing. However, when the plant foods (with their incomplete proteins) are combined with "complementary" foods from other plant groups, the amino acid gap is often bridged.

In a well-balanced diet of vegetables, grains, legumes, and fruits, complete proteins are formed all the time. Whenever beans are combined with rice or lentils with bulgur or corn tossed with beans, complete proteins are formed. When grains are cooked with vegetables, beans are made with pasta, wheat bread is served with bean soup, or a peanut butter sandwich is made with wheat bread, amino acids are combined to form complete proteins. You don't have to be a nutritionist to figure out how to mix and match plant foods to create complete proteins—it happens naturally in the kitchen.

HOW COMPLETE VEGETABLE PROTEINS ARE FORMED

How do plant foods join together to generate complete proteins? Simple: beans are rich in the amino acids tryptophan and lysine but low in methionine. Corn is low in tryptophan and lysine but rich in methionine. When beans and corn are combined in a meal (such as succotash), a complete protein is formed. All 9 essential amino acids are present in the meal, and the body has an available protein to digest.

Of course, some plant foods contain more amino acids than others. Legumes—dried beans, split peas, and lentils—are excellent sources. Soybeans (a legume) are processed into hundreds of protein-rich products available in the marketplace such as tofu, soy milk, tempeh, and miso. (Soy proteins have also shown an ability to reduce cholesterol levels, something no animal protein has ever accomplished.) Whole grains such as quinoa, amaranth, wild rice, brown rice, and seitan (a wheat-based product) are also good sources of amino acids. Nuts and seeds are rich in amino acids as well.

DISCOVER THE VIRTUES OF PLANT PROTEINS: THE RIGHT STUFF

A well-balanced diet of mixed vegetables, grains, fruits, and legumes will supply more than an ample amount of dietary protein. Additionally, plant proteins come with a bonus of complex carbohydrates, fiber, antioxidants, and phytochemicals—the good stuff your body needs to fight disease and enhance your life. Plant foods are also naturally low in saturated fats and cholesterol—the dietary demons that travel with animal proteins.

The purpose of this chapter is not to convert people to a meatless lifestyle—at least not overnight. That would be an unrealistic (even outlandish) agenda. Rather, the goal is to encourage *moderation*, dispel the myths, and expound upon the virtues of plant proteins. (See Table 4.1.)

When meat is on the menu, the best advice is to choose small, well-trimmed portions, and fill up on starches and vegetables. Maybe some day more and more people will feel compelled to slide meat completely *off* the plate—and throw open the door to a healthier, more vibrant lifestyle. But Rome wasn't built in a day.

It all comes down to personal choice. When taking into consideration your overall health and well-being, eating plant foods is the wisest choice you can make. There is a variety of flavorful, nutrient-dense meals that deliver the essential protein and minerals without the heavy baggage of fat. To this end, the recipes in this chapter offer plenty of nutrients—protein, antioxidants, and

For most of America, the first step is to slide meat from the center of the plate to the side. The ultimate aim is to treat meat like a condiment, not the centerpiece, and to pave the way to eating more vegetables, grains, and legumes.

DYNAMIC DUOS   There are myriad ways to create complete proteins by cooking with a variety of plant foods. Here are some suggestions:

- Combine legumes with rice: Cuban black beans and rice, Cajun red beans and rice, Hoppin' John (black-eyed peas and rice), and lentils with rice.
- Combine legumes with grains or pasta: split peas and wild rice, quinoa with black beans, chick-peas with pasta, tabbouleh (bulgur and chick-peas), succotash (beans with corn), veggie-tofu stir-fry with rice, corn tortillas with beans, and pasta fazool.
- Combine legumes with nuts or seeds: three-bean salad with pesto, hummus (chick-peas and sesame seed paste), black bean chili with pumpkin seeds, and sunflower seeds sprinkled over bean or lentil salads.
- Combine grains with dairy products: hot amaranth with milk, whole grain baked goods made with milk, chili or bean soup topped with lowfat yogurt, Indian vegetable curries served with raita (cucumber yogurt sauce), bran cereal with milk, pasta topped with Parmesan cheese, and rice pudding with skim milk.
- Combine grains with seeds or nuts: wheat bread with peanut butter, pesto with pasta, pita with hummus, nutty grain pilafs, and wheat breads with sunflower or sesame seeds.

fiber—but steer clear of animal protein, saturated fats, and dietary cholesterol.

PLANT PROTEINS IN THE KITCHEN

There are a multitude of good sources of protein available in the vegetable kingdom. Protein-rich plant foods offer plenty of pro-

TABLE 4.1
Duel of the Proteins

Animal Proteins	Plant Proteins
Sources include beef, pork, lamb, poultry, dairy (milk), and seafood.	Sources include beans, lentils, split peas, grains, soy milk, and tofu.
Found in foods that are also high in saturated fat and cholesterol.	Found in foods that are lowfat and contain no cholesterol.
Concentrated source of iron and zinc. Dairy products offer calcium.	Well-balanced diet of greens, vegetables, grains, dried fruits, and beans will supply many of the essential minerals, including iron, zinc, and calcium.
Animal food is made of protein and fat. There is no fiber or complex carbohydrates.	Plant foods offer antioxidants, phytochemicals, fiber, and complex carbohydrates.
Animal foods contain plenty of vitamin B-12, which is produced by a bacteria. B-12 is necessary for healthy nerves and maintenance of cells.	Vitamin B-12 is found in tempeh, miso, and fortified cereals, as well as some organic plants. (Ovo-lacto vegetarians can get it from milk, cheese, or yogurt.)
Animal protein contains all nine essential amino acids.	Plant proteins lack one or two amino acids and are "incomplete." When plant foods are combined (rice and beans), complete proteins are formed.
In animal studies, casein (milk protein) raises "bad" cholesterol.	Soy protein can significantly lower bad cholesterol.

tein as well as other healthful phytonutrients, fiber, and complex carbohydrates.

A Cook's Guide to Plant Proteins
Here is a glossary of the many sources of vegetable proteins found in well-stocked grocery stores and natural-health markets.

Amaranth has beige grains shaped like poppy seeds. Cooked amaranth grains have a nutty flavor and creamy texture. The ancient grains were grown centuries ago by the Aztecs and have recently gained a vogue following. Amaranth is high in calcium, iron, and fiber as well as lycine and methionine—amino acids that most other grains lack. It makes a satisfying hot breakfast and thickener for soups and stews and cooks in about 25 minutes. Amaranth also refers to the plant's broad leafy greens with red markings; amaranth greens are cooked like a leafy green vegetable.

Beans are an excellent source of protein, fiber, and complex carbohydrates. The assortment of beans is wide and varied; there are black beans, red kidney beans, small and large white beans, chickpeas, black-eyed peas, and on and on. Almost every country in the world has some type of bean on the menu, from Italian *pasta e fagiola,* Mexican black bean soup, and Jamaican rice and peas to Middle Eastern hummus, Indian dal, and myriad others. (For a complete glossary of beans, turn to Pillar 2: Discover the Goodness of Fiber.)

Lentils come in brown, green, red, and yellow varieties. Lentils have a narrow, oval shape similar to a thin disc or lens. They are staples in Indian, Middle Eastern, North African, and European soups and stews. Most lentils do not require presoaking. (However, soaking old lentils will reduce the cooking time.) Lentils take about 45 minutes to cook; red lentils take slightly less time.

Miso is a thick, fermented paste made with aged soybeans and grains such as barley or rice. Used in Japanese soups, sauces, and dressings, miso is believed to facilitate digestion. The most common forms are barley (red), rice (white), and soy (dark). Miso is available in natural food stores, well-stocked supermarkets, and Asian markets. Miso is a good source of vitamin B-12, an elusive nutrient for some vegetarians.

Quinoa (pronounced "KEEN-wa") is an ancient grain native to the highlands of South America. The grains were grown centuries ago by the Incas and are still known as "the mother grain." Quinoa is considered a protein powerhouse. The tiny beige grains have a ringlike shape and nutty flavor and cook in fifteen to twenty minutes. Rinse quinoa thoroughly before cooking to wash away a natural, soapy-tasting resin called *saponin* that coats the grains. Quinoa is an ideal staple for salads, pilafs, stuffings, thick soups, and side dishes.

Seeds and *Nuts* make excellent "garnishes" for muffins, sweet breads, pancakes, salads, stir-fries, and vegetable medleys. Although nuts and seeds contain plenty of polyunsaturated fat, they also contain vitamin E, selenium, and other healthful micronutrients and amino acids.

Seitan is a wheat product that has been stripped of its starch; the concentrated gluten is left. Seitan is referred to as a meat substitute because of its rich protein density and chewy texture. It is often used in sandwiches, soups, stews, and curries. Look for seitan in the refrigerated section of well-stocked grocery stores and natural food stores.

Soy Foods come in the form of soy burgers, soy breads, soy flour, tofu, textured vegetable protein, and the aforementioned soy milk. There are hundreds of soy products on the shelves. Soy proteins have been shown to lower bad cholesterol (and raise good cholesterol) in people already suffering from high cholesterol.

Soy foods are also brimming with protective phytochemicals such as phytoestrogens, isoflavones, genistein, and saponin, which have been linked with blocking or reversing certain types of cancers. (For more on soy foods, see Pillar 7: On the Trail of Phytochemicals: Vitamins of the Future.)

Soy Milk is a creamy, milklike beverage made from soybeans that have been soaked, mashed, and ground up with water. Soy proteins present in soy milk (along with other natural soy-based substances) have been associated with a reduced risk of certain cancers and lower levels of bad cholesterol. Soy milk can be used like cow's milk: pour it over cereal, add it to baked goods, simmer it in rice pudding and sauces, or blend it with fruit for pseudo milk shakes. For those suffering from lactose intolerance, soy milk is a great alternative to cow's milk.

Spelt may sound like a fad-of-the-month ice cream, but it is an ancient grain. Like amaranth and quinoa, spelt has been cultivated for centuries. Spelt is a lesser-known cousin of wheat and is processed into baking flour, cereals, and an assortment of pastas including elbow macaroni, spaghetti, and shells. Spelt pasta has a dark color and grainy flavor; it cooks just like Italian semolina pasta. Although more expensive than Italian pasta, spelt pasta is well worth a try.

Split Peas are whole green or yellow peas that have been split along a natural break. Split peas cook to a puréed consistency and are a favorite ingredient in thick European soups and stews. To optimize the protein content, add brown rice, barley, or wild rice to long-cooking split pea soups. Split peas take one to two hours to cook, but patience is a virtue. Like old lentils, split peas should be soaked ahead of time if they are old.

Tempeh is a chewy meat substitute made from cooked and aged soybeans. Often sold as rectangular patties, tempeh can be sliced or cubed and added to sandwiches, stews, or soups. Tempeh can also be grilled or stir-fried. Popular in Indonesian cooking, tempeh is sold in the refrigerated section of natural food stores and in well-stocked supermarkets. Add tempeh to hearty chili or vegetable stew, stir-fries, and red sauces for pasta.

Tofu is a versatile soybean product with a rather bland taste. Also called bean curd, it is often sold as a white square block packaged in water. The texture varies from extra firm and firm to soft and silken (which has the texture of thick pudding). Tofu can be grilled, stir-fried, baked, and added to soups, salads, pilafs, and red sauces. It also can be used in cheesecakes and fruit shakes.

Tofu must be stored in a small tub of water, and it is a good idea to change the water on a daily basis. After a package of tofu is opened, it has a shelf life of about four to five days. It is best to cook or blanch tofu before eating; a natural bacteria coating tofu can cause digestive problems in some people. Like other soy foods, tofu comes with a panoply of protective phytonutrients that fight cancer and bad cholesterol. (For more on tofu, see Pillar 7: On the Trail of Phytochemicals: Vitamins of the Future.)

SIGNATURE RECIPES FOR THE PROTEIN-RICH, HEALTHY DIET

Maple Amaranth with Wheat Germ

Japanese Noodle Soup with Tofu

Succotash Bisque

Quinoa Tabbouleh

Tropical Black Bean and Rice Salad

Confetti Quinoa Salad with Lime

Two-Bean, Corn, and Artichoke Salad

Power Pasta Salad with Chick-Peas

Black Bean Succotash

Sizzling Black Bean–Tofu Chili

Tofu and Veggie Rice Toss

Middle Eastern Lentil, Spinach, and Bulgur Stew

Savory Lentils with Baby Squash

Red Bean Ratatouille Stew

Yellow Rice and Black Beans

Veggie, Rice, and Bean Burrito

Mashed Potatoes with Soy Milk

Super Grain Cornbread

Blueberry-Banana Soy Shake

Fruity Soy Rice Pudding

Additional health benefits are noted with each recipe.

Maple Amaranth with Wheat Germ

This delicious hot breakfast (or late-night snack) is reminiscent of oatmeal. Amaranth has a nutty flavor and creamy texture.

1 cup amaranth
2 tablespoons real maple syrup
2 tablespoons wheat germ

In a medium saucepan combine the amaranth and 3 cups water and bring to a simmer. Cook for 20 to 25 minutes over medium-low heat, stirring occasionally, until the grains become thick and soft.

Spoon the amaranth into bowls and swirl in the maple syrup. Sprinkle the wheat germ over the top. Serve at once.

YIELD: 3 TO 4 SERVINGS

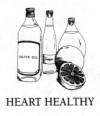

HEART HEALTHY

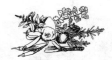

FIRE AND SPICE

POWER EATING

HELPFUL HINT

For additional nutrients and flavor, add diced fruit (such as apples, pears, or peaches) to the simmering amaranth.

Japanese Noodle Soup with Tofu

ANTIOXIDANTS

HEART HEALTHY

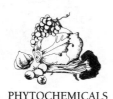

PHYTOCHEMICALS

This brothy noodle soup is abundant with vegetables and aromatic flavors.

2 teaspoons peanut oil
2 carrots, sliced at an angle
2 cloves garlic, minced
1 teaspoon minced ginger root
5 cups vegetable broth
2 cups coarsely chopped bok choy
2 large scallions, chopped
1/4 pound extra-firm tofu, diced
2 or 3 radishes, thinly sliced
2 to 3 tablespoons low-sodium soy sauce
1/2 teaspoon black pepper
8 to 10 ounces Japanese noodles (soba or udon)
2 tablespoons miso paste
2 ounces mung bean sprouts

In a large saucepan heat the oil over medium-high heat. Add the carrots, garlic, and ginger and cook, stirring, for 2 minutes. Add the broth, bok choy, scallions, tofu, radishes, soy sauce, and black pepper and bring to a simmer. Cook over medium heat for about 10 minutes, stirring occasionally.

In another large saucepan bring 3 quarts of water to a boil over medium-high heat. Place the noodles in the boiling water, stir, and return to a boil. Cook for 6 to 8 minutes until al dente, stirring occasionally. Drain the pasta in a colander.

Meanwhile, dissolve the miso paste in 2 to 3 tablespoons warm water. At the last minute, stir the miso paste mixture into the soup and cook for about 1 minute more. *Do not boil* once the miso has been added.

Using tongs, place the cooked noodles in large soup bowls. Ladle the miso soup over the noodles. Sprinkle the sprouts over the top.

YIELD: 4 TO 6 SERVINGS

HELPFUL HINT

Japanese noodles and miso can be found in Asian markets and well-stocked grocery stores. Varieties of miso include barley miso (also called red), rice miso (white), and soy miso (dark). Chicken or fish stock may be used in place of vegetable broth.

Succotash Bisque

This satisfying bisque has a little of everything—legumes, rice, corn, peppers, and carrots. Its soothing, porridgelike texture calls to mind a hearty split pea soup.

ANTIOXIDANTS

HEART HEALTHY

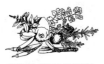

FIRE AND SPICE

1 tablespoon canola oil
2 carrots, diced
1 medium yellow onion, diced
1 green bell pepper, seeded and diced
2 or 3 cloves garlic, minced
4 cups vegetable broth or water
2 cups green lima beans (10-ounce frozen package)
1½ cups corn kernels, fresh or frozen
¼ cup long grain white rice
1 tablespoon dried parsley
2 teaspoons dried oregano
½ teaspoon salt
½ teaspoon black pepper

In a large saucepan heat the oil over high heat. Add the carrots, onion, bell pepper, and garlic and cook, stirring, for 5 to 7 minutes over medium-high heat. Add the broth or water, lima beans, corn, rice, parsley, oregano, salt, and pepper. Cook over medium-low heat for about 20 minutes, stirring occasionally.

Transfer the soup (in batches) to a food processor fitted with a steel blade or to a blender and process for 5 to 10 seconds until puréed. Return the soup to the pan and bring to a simmer.

Ladle the soup into bowls and serve hot.

YIELD: 6 SERVINGS

Quinoa Tabbouleh

*This "wheat garden salad" of Middle Eastern origin is reinvented with
quinoa, a protein-rich supergrain from South America.*

1 cup bulgur or cracked wheat
1¹/₂ cups boiling water
¹/₂ cup quinoa, rinsed
2 or 3 large scallions, chopped
¹/₂ cup chopped parsley
2 tablespoons chopped mint
1 large tomato, diced
1 cucumber, peeled and chopped
Juice of 1¹/₂ to 2 lemons
2 tablespoons olive oil
¹/₂ teaspoon black pepper
¹/₂ teaspoon salt

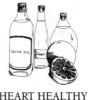

HEART HEALTHY

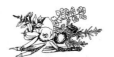

FIRE AND SPICE

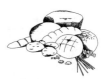

POWER EATING

Combine the bulgur and boiling water in a pan, cover, and let
stand for 20 minutes until most of the water is absorbed. Drain
any excess liquid.

Meanwhile, in a small saucepan combine the quinoa and 1 cup
water and bring to a simmer. Cover and cook for 13 to 15 minutes
over medium-low heat until all of the water is absorbed. Fluff the
grains and set aside for 10 minutes.

In a mixing bowl, combine the remaining ingredients and toss
thoroughly. Fold in the bulgur and quinoa. Refrigerate the salad
for 1 to 2 hours before serving.

Serve the tabbouleh over a bed of leafy greens with warm pita
bread on the side.

YIELD: 4 TO 6 SERVINGS

Tropical Black Bean and Rice Salad

FIBER

HEART HEALTHY

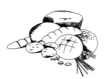

POWER EATING

Black beans and rice are natural companions. Here the two staples combine with lime, cilantro, vegetables, and herbs.

2 cans (15 ounces each) black beans, drained
2 cups cooked long grain white or brown rice
4 whole scallions, chopped
2 tomatoes, diced
1 cucumber, peeled and diced
1 large jalapeño pepper, seeded and minced (optional)
2 tablespoons canola oil
Juice of 1 or 2 limes
2 tablespoons chopped fresh cilantro
2 teaspoons dried oregano
$^1/_2$ teaspoon ground cumin
$^1/_2$ teaspoon black pepper
$^1/_2$ teaspoon salt

In a large mixing bowl combine all of the ingredients and mix thoroughly. Chill for about 1 hour to allow the flavors to meld together. Serve over a bed of leafy green lettuce.

YIELD: 6 SERVINGS

HELPFUL HINT

If cilantro is unavailable, add about $^1/_4$ cup chopped fresh parsley.

Confetti Quinoa Salad with Lime

Light and healthful, this colorful salad makes a satisfying side dish or first course.

- 1 cup quinoa, rinsed
- 1 can (15 ounces) red kidney beans, drained
- 4 whole scallions, chopped
- 1 red bell pepper, seeded and diced
- 1 jalapeño pepper, seeded and minced
- 1 can (14 ounces) corn kernels, drained
- 1 tablespoon canola oil
- 2 tablespoons chopped parsley
- $1/2$ teaspoon black pepper
- $1/2$ teaspoon salt
- 2 limes, cut into wedges

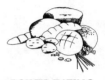

In a medium saucepan combine the quinoa and 2 cups water and bring to a simmer. Cover and cook for 15 minutes over medium heat until all of the liquid is absorbed. Fluff the grains and set aside for 5 minutes.

Meanwhile in a medium mixing bowl combine the beans, scallions, bell peppers, jalapeño, corn, oil, parsley, pepper, and salt. Blend in the cooked quinoa and squeeze half of the limes into the salad. Serve the salad warm or chill for later.

Squeeze the remaining lime over the top just before serving.

YIELD: 4 SERVINGS

FIBER

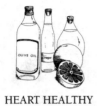

HEART HEALTHY

Two-Bean, Corn, and Artichoke Salad

This quick-and-easy salad is brimming with fiber and protein. Balsamic vinegar adds a smooth, mellow flavor.

1 can (15 ounces) chick-peas, drained
1 can (15 ounces) red kidney beans or black-eyed peas, drained
1 can (14 ounces) artichoke hearts, rinsed and coarsely chopped
4 whole scallions, trimmed and chopped
2 large tomatoes, diced
1 cup cooked corn kernels
3 or 4 cloves garlic, minced
2 tablespoons olive oil or canola oil
2 to 3 tablespoons balsamic vinegar
1/4 cup chopped fresh parsley
2 teaspoons dried oregano
1/2 teaspoon black pepper
1/2 teaspoon salt

Combine all of the ingredients in a large mixing bowl and blend well. Refrigerate the salad for 30 minutes to 1 hour to allow the flavors to meld together. (The salad may be made up to a day ahead of serving time.)

When ready, serve the salad over a bed of leaf lettuce.

YIELD: 6 SERVINGS

Power Pasta Salad with Chick-Peas

Pasta and beans are a classic protein combination.

FIBER

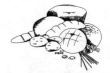

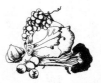

POWER EATING

1/4 cup canola oil

3 tablespoons balsamic vinegar

1 1/2 teaspoons Dijon-style mustard

1 teaspoon dried oregano

1/2 teaspoon dried basil

1/2 teaspoon thyme

1/2 teaspoon black pepper

1/2 teaspoon salt

1/4 cup chopped fresh basil or parsley (optional)

8 ounces cooked pasta spirals or radiatore

1 can (15 ounces) chick-peas, drained

4 whole scallions, chopped

1 yellow or green bell pepper, seeded and diced

2 tomatoes, diced

2 large cloves garlic, minced

1/4 cup grated Parmesan cheese

PHYTOCHEMICALS

To make the dressing, combine the oil, vinegar, mustard, oregano, dried basil, thyme, pepper, salt, and fresh basil or parsley in a mixing bowl and whisk thoroughly. (Or combine in a jar with a lid and shake well.) Refrigerate for 15 to 30 minutes to allow the flavors to meld together.

In a large mixing bowl blend the vinaigrette dressing with the cooked pasta and remaining ingredients. Serve at once or refrigerate for later.

YIELD: 4 SERVINGS

Black Bean Succotash

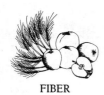

FIBER

HEART HEALTHY

Black beans give this colorful Native American dish a Southwestern personality.

1 tablespoon canola oil
1 small onion, finely chopped
1 red or green bell pepper, seeded and diced
2 cloves garlic, minced
2 cups corn kernels, fresh or frozen
1 can (15 ounces) black beans, drained
1 teaspoon dried oregano
$^{1}/_{2}$ teaspoon black pepper
$^{1}/_{2}$ teaspoon salt
2 large scallions, chopped
2 to 3 tablespoons minced fresh cilantro

In a medium saucepan heat the oil over medium-high heat. Add the onion, bell pepper, and garlic and cook, stirring, for 5 to 6 minutes. Add the corn, beans, oregano, pepper, and salt and cook for 6 to 8 minutes more over medium heat, stirring occasionally, until the vegetables and beans are steaming. Blend in the scallions and cilantro. Serve at once.

YIELD: 4 SERVINGS

HELPFUL HINT

This can accompany a traditional chicken or seafood entrée.

Sizzling Black Bean–Tofu Chili

Two protein superstars, beans and tofu, come together in this robust chili.

FIBER

1 tablespoon canola oil
1 medium yellow onion, diced
1 green bell pepper, seeded and diced
2 celery stalks, chopped
2 or 3 cloves garlic, minced
1 can (28 ounces) crushed tomatoes
1 can (15 ounces) black beans, drained
$^1/_2$ pound extra-firm tofu, diced, or $^1/_4$ pound seitan, diced
1 tablespoon chili powder
1 tablespoon dried parsley
1 tablespoon dried oregano
2 teaspoons ground cumin
$^1/_2$ teaspoon black pepper
$^1/_2$ teaspoon salt
Plain lowfat yogurt (optional)

HEART HEALTHY

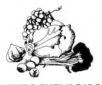

PHYTOCHEMICALS

In a large saucepan heat the oil. Add the onion, bell pepper, celery, and garlic and cook, stirring, over medium-high heat for 5 to 7 minutes. Stir in the crushed tomatoes, beans, $^1/_2$ cup water, the tofu or seitan, chili powder, parsley, oregano, cumin, pepper, and salt. Cook for 20 to 25 minutes (uncovered) over medium-low heat, stirring occasionally.

Remove the chili from the heat and let stand for 5 to 10 minutes before serving. Serve with warm bread and a few dollops of lowfat yogurt (in place of the traditional full-fat sour cream).

YIELD: 6 SERVINGS

Tofu and Veggie Rice Toss

HEART HEALTHY

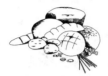

POWER EATING

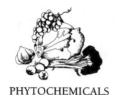

PHYTOCHEMICALS

This unpretentious dish is prepared like fried rice (only without meat and with less oil). Tofu supplies texture and substance in lieu of shredded meat and eggs.

1 tablespoon canola oil
10 to 12 button mushrooms, sliced
1 medium red bell pepper, seeded and diced
1 medium red onion, diced
1 jalapeño pepper, seeded and minced (optional)
1/2 pound extra-firm tofu, diced
4 cups cooked long grain brown rice or basmati rice
2 to 3 tablespoons low-sodium soy sauce
1 1/2 teaspoons toasted sesame oil
3 to 4 tablespoons chopped parsley

In a large skillet or wok heat the oil over medium-high heat. Add the mushrooms, bell pepper, onion, and jalapeño (if desired). Cook, stirring, for about 3 minutes. Stir in the tofu and sauté for about 5 minutes more, until the vegetables are tender. Stir in the rice, soy sauce, and sesame oil and reduce the heat to medium. Cook, stirring frequently, until the rice is steaming.

Spoon the rice-and-tofu mixture onto serving plates and sprinkle the parsley over the top.

YIELD: 4 SERVINGS

HELPFUL HINT

Add 1 tablespoon minced ginger root along with the vegetables. Zucchini, corn, broccoli, or snow peas can also be included in the stir-fry. If desired, 1/2 pound of chicken (cut in strips) or shellfish can also be added.

Middle Eastern Lentil, Spinach, and Bulgur Stew

ANTIOXIDANTS

This pot of legumes and grains provides plenty of protein, fiber, and get-up-and-go fuel.

1 cup dried brown lentils, rinsed
1/2 cup coarse bulgur
1/2 teaspoon salt
1/2 teaspoon black pepper
2 cups chopped fresh spinach
1 to 2 tablespoons olive oil
1 medium yellow onion, slivered

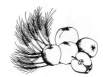

FIBER

In a medium saucepan combine the lentils and 4 1/2 cups water and bring to a simmer over medium heat. Cook for about 25 minutes, stirring occasionally. Stir in the bulgur, salt, and pepper and cook for 15 to 20 minutes more over medium-low heat, stirring occasionally, until the lentils are tender. (Add a little hot water if necessary.) Stir in the spinach, cover, and set aside for about 10 minutes.

HEART HEALTHY

In another skillet heat the oil. Add the onion and cook, stirring, for 7 to 9 minutes until the onions are lightly browned. Stir the onions into the lentil and bulgur stew. Serve with warm pita bread.

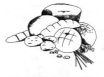

POWER EATING

YIELD: 3 TO 4 SERVINGS

HELPFUL HINT

For a tangy version, squeeze 1 or 2 lemons over the stew before serving. If desired, the stew can be served with traditional chicken or fish entrées.

Savory Lentils with Baby Squash

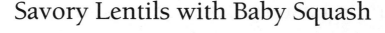

Young zucchini and patty pan squash add a newfangled twist to this hearty cauldron of lentils and vegetables.

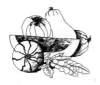
ANTIOXIDANTS

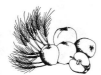
FIBER

HEART HEALTHY

POWER EATING

1 tablespoon canola oil
1 medium yellow onion, diced
1 large stalk celery, chopped
4 cloves garlic, minced
1 cup green lentils, rinsed
2 cups diced sweet potatoes or butternut squash (peeled)
1 teaspoon ground cumin
1 teaspoon ground coriander
$^1/_2$ teaspoon black pepper
10 to 12 baby patty pan squash or baby zucchini
$^1/_4$ cup chopped fresh parsley
$^3/_4$ teaspoon salt

In a large saucepan heat the oil over medium heat. Add the onion, celery, and garlic and cook, stirring, for 5 minutes. Stir in 7 cups water and the lentils and bring to a simmer. Cook for 10 minutes over medium heat, stirring occasionally. Stir in the sweet potatoes, cumin, coriander, and pepper and cook for 10 minutes more. Stir in the baby squash and cook about 15 minutes more until the lentils are tender. Stir in the parsley and salt; let stand for 5 to 10 minutes before serving.

Ladle the stew into bowls and serve with warm whole wheat tortillas.

YIELD: 6 SERVINGS

Red Bean Ratatouille Stew

Adding beans to ratatouille is an easy and flavorful way to increase the protein and fiber content. Serve the vegetable stew over pasta and rice.

ANTIOXIDANTS

2 tablespoons canola oil
1 medium yellow onion, diced
1 green bell pepper, seeded and diced
8 ounces button mushrooms, sliced
2 cups diced eggplant
4 cloves garlic, minced
1 can (14 ounces) stewed tomatoes
1 can (14 ounces) tomato purée
1 can (14 ounces) red kidney beans, drained
1 tablespoon dried parsley
2 teaspoons dried oregano
$1/2$ teaspoon black pepper
$1/2$ teaspoon salt

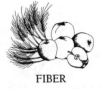

FIBER

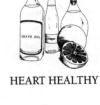

HEART HEALTHY

In a large saucepan heat the oil over medium heat. Add the onion, bell pepper, mushrooms, eggplant, and garlic and cook, stirring, for 8 to 10 minutes over medium heat until the vegetables are tender. Stir in the stewed tomatoes, tomato purée, beans, parsley, oregano, pepper, and salt and cook over medium-low heat for 15 minutes, stirring occasionally.

Remove from the heat. Serve the ratatouille over pasta or rice in shallow bowls.

YIELD: 4 SERVINGS

PHYTOCHEMICALS

Yellow Rice and Black Beans

FIBER

This vibrant pilaf of beans and rice is fortified with orzo, a rice-shaped pasta.

HEART HEALTHY

1   tablespoon olive oil
1   medium yellow onion, chopped
2   cloves garlic, minced
1   cup long grain white rice or parboiled rice
$1/2$ cup orzo pasta
$1/2$ teaspoon salt
$1/2$ teaspoon black pepper
$1/4$ teaspoon ground turmeric
1   can (15 ounces) black beans, drained
$1/4$ cup chopped fresh parsley

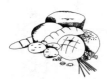

POWER EATING

In a medium saucepan heat the oil over medium heat. Add the onion and garlic and cook, stirring, for 3 to 4 minutes. Stir in the rice, orzo, salt, pepper, and turmeric and cook for 1 minute more over low heat, stirring frequently. Stir in $2^{1}/2$ cups water and the black beans and bring to a simmer. (Add $1/4$ cup additional water if using parboiled rice.) Cover and cook for 15 to 18 minutes over low heat.

Remove from the heat, fluff the rice, and fold in the parsley. Let stand for 10 minutes before serving.

YIELD: 4 SERVINGS

HELPFUL HINT

Orzo, also called rosa marina, can be found in the pasta section of supermarkets and natural food stores.

Veggie, Rice, and Bean Burrito

Gourmet burritos filled with beans and rice have become part of the nation's grand culinary melting pot.

ANTIOXIDANTS

1   tablespoon canola oil
8 to 10 button mushrooms, sliced
1   red bell pepper, seeded and diced
2   cloves garlic, minced
2   cups cooked brown rice or white rice
1   can (15 ounces) red kidney beans or black beans, drained
1   can (11 ounces) corn, drained
4   scallions, chopped
$1/2$ teaspoon ground cumin
$1/2$ teaspoon black pepper
4   flour tortillas (10 inches in diameter)
$1/2$ cup shredded reduced-fat Swiss or Monterey jack cheese
$1/2$ cup prepared salsa

FIBER

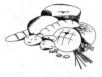

POWER EATING

In a large non-stick skillet heat the oil over medium-high heat. Add the mushrooms, bell pepper, and garlic and cook, stirring, for 5 to 6 minutes. Stir in the rice, beans, corn, scallions, cumin, and pepper and cook for 4 to 6 minutes over medium heat, stirring frequently, until the mixture is steaming. Remove from the heat.

Warm the tortillas over a hot burner or pan and place on large serving plates. Spoon the rice and bean mixture down the center of each tortilla. Top each with 2 tablespoons of cheese and roll the tortillas around the filling (creating burritos). Spoon your favorite salsa over the top of the burritos.

YIELD: 4 SERVINGS

Mashed Potatoes with Soy Milk

HEART HEALTHY

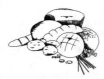

POWER EATING

For this wholesome bowl of mashed potatoes, protein-rich soy milk makes a nutritious substitute for heavy cream, milk, and butter.

4 cups diced white potatoes (scrubbed, not peeled)
1/2 cup soy milk
1/4 cup chopped fresh parsley
1/2 teaspoon salt
1/4 teaspoon white pepper
2 large whole scallions, chopped

In a medium saucepan bring 2½ quarts of water to a boil. Place the potatoes in the boiling water and cook for 18 to 20 minutes until easily pierced with a fork. Drain in a colander.

Transfer the potatoes to a medium mixing bowl. Add the soy milk, parsley, salt, and pepper to the potatoes and mash with the back of a spoon or potato masher until puréed. Transfer to a serving bowl and sprinkle the scallions over the top.

YIELD: 4 SERVINGS

Super Grain Cornbread

With a little creativity, ordinary cornbread is transformed into an extraordinary treat fortified with nutrient-rich quinoa.

HEART HEALTHY

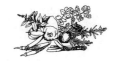

FIRE AND SPICE

$^1/_2$ cup quinoa, rinsed
1 cup yellow cornmeal
1 cup unbleached all-purpose flour
$^1/_3$ cup sugar
1 tablespoon baking powder
$^1/_2$ teaspoon salt
1 large egg plus 1 egg white, beaten
1 cup lowfat milk or soy milk
$^1/_3$ cup canola oil
2 tablespoons chopped pimientos (optional)
1 cup corn kernels, fresh or frozen and thawed

In a small saucepan combine the quinoa and 1 cup water and bring to a simmer. Cover and cook for 13 to 15 minutes over medium-low heat, until all of the water is absorbed. Remove from the heat and fluff the grains. Set aside for 10 to 15 minutes and let cool.

Meanwhile, preheat the oven to 375 degrees F.

In a medium mixing bowl, combine the cornmeal, flour, sugar, baking powder, and salt. In a separate bowl, whisk together the eggs, milk, oil, pimientos, and corn. Gently fold the liquid ingredients into the dry ingredients until the mixture forms a batter. Fold in the cooked quinoa.

Pour the batter into a lightly greased 9-inch-round, deep-dish baking pan. Bake for 20 to 25 minutes, until the crust is lightly browned and a toothpick inserted in the center comes out clean. Remove the cornbread from the oven and let cool for a few minutes. Cut into wedges and serve warm.

YIELD: 8 TO 10 SERVINGS

Blueberry-Banana Soy Shake

HEART HEALTHY

The next time you crave ice cream, try this delicious and naturally sweet treat. Protein-rich soy milk adds creamy texture to bananas and blueberries.

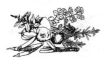

FIRE AND SPICE

2 cups soy milk
2 cups blueberries (thawed, if frozen)
2 bananas, sliced
2 tablespoons wheat germ (optional)

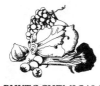

PHYTOCHEMICALS

Combine all of the ingredients in a blender and process for 5 to 10 seconds until creamy. Pour into cold glasses and serve as a beverage or dessert.

YIELD: 2 SERVINGS

Fruity Soy Rice Pudding

Rice pudding is a good dessert to incorporate health-promoting staples such as apples, dried apricots, raisins, and soy milk.

FIBER

2½ cups cooked short grain rice (preferably arborio)
1½ cups soy milk
1 red apple, diced
⅓ cup brown sugar
½ cup dried apricots, chopped
¼ cup raisins
½ teaspoon ground nutmeg

HEART HEALTHY

In a medium saucepan combine all of the ingredients except the nutmeg. Cook for 10 to 12 minutes over medium-low heat, stirring frequently. Remove from the heat and let cool slightly. Chill for at least 1 hour before serving.

When ready to serve, spoon the pudding into bowls and sprinkle the nutmeg over the top.

YIELD: 4 SERVINGS

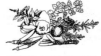

FIRE AND SPICE

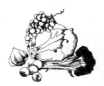

PHYTOCHEMICALS

HELPFUL HINT

For 2½ cups of cooked arborio rice, combine 1 cup of rice with 3 cups water and cook, stirring often, for 22 to 25 minutes over medium heat.

FIRE AND SPICE:
High-Flavor, Low-Sodium Cooking with Herbs, Spices, and Chili Peppers

Y EARS AGO, THE TYPICAL AMERICAN CUPBOARD CON-
tained all of two spices, salt and pepper. Go up to an attic (or
garage sale) and dust off an old cookbook and you'll uncover
recipes loaded with butter, cream, lard, and lots of salt. Herbs and
exotic spices were rarely mentioned. Chili peppers and hot sauces
were unheard of. Unlike ethnic cuisines (which were spicy and intense), the traditional American triad of meat, potatoes, and vegetables was bland, predictable, and remarkably free of spices.

Then came the culinary revolution of the 1980s. First there was
pesto tortellini, an herb-scented dish coated with an Italian herbal
paste. Pesto tortellini became all the rage at restaurants, gourmet
take-out delis, and homes with sophisticated tastes. The fragrant
blend of fresh basil, garlic, nuts, and Parmesan cheese was
blended, folded, and spread into everything from pizza and pasta

to salad dressings, soups, breads, dips, and marinades. As the aroma of pesto swept over the country, America's taste buds were liberated from the dreary and the mundane.

At about the same time a wave of Thai, Vietnamese, Caribbean, Cajun, Southwestern, and Pan-African restaurants appeared from coast to coast. The rise of ethnic restaurants emboldened cooks to prepare high-spirited dishes at home with cilantro, jalapeño peppers, ginger, curry powder, lemon grass, and other exotic flavorings. Soon a variety of piquant salsas, sour chutneys, pungent Indian curries, soothing black bean soups, and tart vinaigrettes appeared on restaurant menus and dining room tables across the land. The gates to a more adventurous culinary era had swung open.

The recent culinary renaissance ushered in a greater appreciation for assertive flavors provided by herbs, spices, and chili peppers. Fresh cilantro, basil, dill, and mint are no longer the exclusive province of gardeners and gourmet chefs and have become available throughout the year (and positively copious in the summer and fall). Potent spices such as cumin, coriander, cloves, and curry powder have leapt from ethnic pantries to mainstream kitchens. The demand for piquant chili peppers, hot sauces, and spicy seasonings has flourished.

This reinvigoration of the American palate bodes well for disciples of healthy cooking. Herbs, spices, and chili peppers contain virtually zero calories, sodium, or fat. Their bold and distinctive presence also reduces the need for adding salt, cream, or butter to a meal. With so many vibrant and diverse tastes to excite our appetite, there is little need to reach for the old salt shaker.

Unfortunately, despite the epicurean explosion of interesting flavors and adventurous tastes, there is still too much sodium (i.e., salt) in the typical Western diet. Much of the population is hooked on salt. Although the issue of sodium does not seem to generate the same electricity as other dietary villains, such as saturated fat and cholesterol, there is much evidence associating high-sodium diets with hypertension (high blood pressure). Hypertension is a significant piece in the ongoing puzzle of what causes heart attacks and heart disease.

THE TANGLED WEB OF SODIUM, SALT, AND HYPERTENSION

Sodium is an omnipresent substance found in almost all of the foods we eat. It occurs naturally in plant foods and is unmercifully added to just about every kind of processed food imaginable. From snack foods, tomato juice, canned vegetables and soups and cured meats to commercial breads, cereals, salad dressings, soy sauce, and cheeses, sodium is everywhere. Fast foods and prepared meals are loaded with sodium. The mineral is one of the most common additives in the nation's food supply.

Although the terms *sodium* and *table salt* are often used interchangeably, they are not exactly the same entity. Table salt is composed of sodium chloride (a chemical compound), which is about 40 percent sodium. Just as sodium is a prevalent additive in many processed foods, salt is a major fixture in home-cooked meals. It is not unusual for people to reach for the salt shaker before tasting the food on their plate. Adding salt to foods has become an unconscious habit, like reaching for butter when dinner rolls arrive.

Americans have a penchant for salty foods. The typical diet contains an excess of sodium; it has been estimated that we consume *10 to 35 times* more sodium than our bodies need. (The body's requirement for salt is less than ⅛ teaspoon per day.) If this excessive sodium intake did not pose a health problem, it could be written off as a cultural quirk. Unfortunately, there is a connection between sodium intake and blood pressure (albeit a controversial connection). High-salt diets in some individuals can lead to hypertension (another name for high blood pressure). Hypertension is considered a cardinal precursor to heart attack, stroke, and other heart-related disorders.

AN IN-DEPTH LOOK AT BLOOD PRESSURE AND HYPERTENSION

Blood pressure is medically defined as the pressure exerted by the blood against the arterial walls. The heart exerts this pressure as it pumps blood through the arteries. Blood pressure is expressed as a ratio of two numbers, such as 120/80, which happens to be a normal reading. The upper number, called *systolic pressure*, measures the pressure exerted against the arterial walls when the heart is pumping. The lower number, called *diastolic pressure*, measures the pressure of the arterial walls when the heart is resting between beats. Blood pressure is influenced by a variety of factors, including family medical history, smoking, frequency of exercise, and diet.

Hypertension occurs when the blood pressure exceeds 140/90. Hypertension is a cardinal risk factor for heart disease, stroke, and kidney disease. When hypertension is combined with other risk factors such as high levels of bad cholesterol, overweight, and a sedentary lifestyle, the risk of heart disease rises even more.

THE GREAT DEBATE: TO SALT OR NOT TO SALT?

The relationship between hypertension and heart disease has been firmly established in the medical community. The controversy arises when sodium enters the equation. Is there a connection between sodium and hypertension? Most nutritionists think so. Generally speaking, most nutritionists believe that there is a strong correlation between a high-salt diet and hypertension.

A preponderance of studies have linked high-salt diets with the occurrence of hypertension. Numerous animal studies and clinical studies on humans have concluded that a high salt intake is associated with high blood pressure and low salt intake is associated with low blood pressure. This connection is reaffirmed in population studies around the world. Populations with high-salt diets have higher blood pressures than populations known for lower salt consumption. In cultures where little salt is eaten, hypertension is a relatively rare occurrence.

On the other hand, there are reasonable professionals who strongly disagree about the role salt plays in preventing or controlling hypertension. The Salt Institute, an industry trade group, points to conflicting results produced by a pool of blood pressure studies called the Intersalt study. The Salt Institute argues that reducing dietary salt will have negligible impact on the general population's health and well-being. Another controversial report (backed by Campbell Soup) grabbed headlines by questioning the wisdom of restricting salt intake as a means to lowering blood pressure. Although many news reports seemed to exult in this apparent liberation of salt from the specter of "unhealthy pleasures," the report was roundly criticized by health experts for its myopic interpretations.

Needless to say, the salt controversy is far from being settled. So who—and what—do you believe? It is a good idea to examine your own current health condition. People already suffering from hypertension are more likely to be sensitive to dietary sodium than those with normal or low blood pressure. Depending on your family history and lifestyle, you may (or may not) be prone to developing hypertension. However, if you do not have hypertension today, it does not necessarily mean you are set for life. Blood pressure almost universally creeps upward as you grow older. Overall, approximately one in three Americans is believed to suffer from hypertension—and many is not aware of it.

THE URGE TO PURGE: WAYS TO REDUCE THE SALT IN YOUR DIET

Ultimately, the detection and proper treatment for hypertension and borderline high blood pressure is best left in the hands of your doctor. Prescriptive drugs with minimal side effects have been deployed for decades in the battle to control high blood pressure. Reducing the amount of dietary sodium is one aspect of treatment. In general, it is easy to avoid high-sodium foods if your diet is centered on vegetables, fruits, grains, and legumes.

It is advisable to keep your dietary sodium in check. When reducing the salt in your diet, the operative word is *moderation*. A palate accustomed to salty foods might find low-sodium foods rather bland. Conversely, the reduction of salt should be correlated with an increased usage of herbs, spices, and chilies. Believe it or not, there is a universe of assertive flavors that will make salt seem positively boring and trite.

A Matter of Taste

Speaking from a culinary perspective, salt is overused and abused. If a dish is lacking verve, the easy way out is to reach for the salt shaker. Faced with a dish that is "missing something," salt becomes a crutch. Too much salt can steamroll over other flavors and obliterate any subtle nuances. Eventually all salty foods start tasting alike. Food becomes boring.

Few people suggest that salt should be banished from the kitchen. When used in moderation, salt enhances and heightens the potency of a dish and wakes up sleepy flavors. However, the world of herbs, spices, and chili peppers occupies a far greater role in the grand culinary mosaic. Salt has a tiny corner in the big picture. (When it comes to baking, salt is an important leavening agent in breads and baked goods.)

Remember, moderation is the key. Going cold turkey on salt almost never works. Out of the blue my grandmother started baking bread without salt. Her legendary fresh bread soon tasted flat and floury, a pale imitation of her original bread. The no-sodium bread caused disappointment and nearly tore the family asunder. Besieged, she reverted to her original recipe with a slightly reduced salt content, and then everyone was happy.

EIGHTEEN TIPS FOR REDUCING DIETARY SODIUM (AND CONTROLLING YOUR BLOOD PRESSURE)

In general, the prevalence of processed foods—canned goods, cured meats, fast foods, cheese, and so forth—is responsible for the excessive sodium intake found in most American diets. Here are a few suggestions to reduce the amount of sodium intake in the typical meal plan.

1. Throw away the salt shaker sitting on the dining room table. Store the salt in the kitchen and reserve it for cooking uses only.
2. Avoid using bouillon cubes, canned broths, soup bases, and commercial dressings. Many brands are atrociously high in sodium, MSG, and fat.
3. Avoid cooking with garlic salt, onion salt, celery salt, and other sodium-enhanced spices. If you own these spices, throw them out.
4. Read the labels of commercial spice blends (such as blackened seasoning, Jamaican jerk spices, and chili powder). Avoid brands in which salt is a main ingredient.
5. Stock up on dried herbs and spices. Every heart-healthy spice cabinet should contain a variety of seasonings such as oregano, thyme, basil, cumin, curry powder, chili powder, nutmeg, allspice, and paprika.
6. Add fresh herbs to the shopping list (such as parsley, basil, cilantro, chives, and mint). Sprinkle fresh herbs over a dish at the last minute.
7. Cook with low-sodium soy sauce without any added monosodium glutamate.
8. To perk up low-sodium soups and sauces, add a squeeze of fresh lemon or wine vinegar at the last minute.
9. Include the indispensable trio of garlic, ginger root, and chili peppers. Think of these assertive ingredients as necessary pantry staples, not as exotic artifacts.

10. Limit your consumption of fast foods, which tend to be high in sodium (and fat). If you are addicted to french fries and hash browns, request salt-free alternatives.

11. Restrict your consumption of salty nuts, crackers, popcorn, and pretzels.

12. Avoid eating cured meats, luncheon meats, bacon, sardines, and anchovies—all high in sodium.

13. Whenever possible, choose low-sodium canned vegetables and beans (corn kernels, beans, and stewed tomatoes).

14. Cook beans and lentils from scratch once in a while. Canned beans are convenient and easy to use, but, like other canned products, they contain added salt.

15. In general, cook with fresh and frozen vegetables more than canned vegetables; canned vegetables often contain more salt than their less processed counterparts.

16. Eat more of such potassium-rich foods as bananas, figs, potatoes, cantaloupe, beans, oranges, and orange juice. Potassium, along with sodium and calcium, helps regulate the body fluids.

17. Exercise regularly. People with sedentary lifestyles (couch potatoes) are more likely to suffer from high blood pressure than active people who bicycle, jog, take brisk walks, jump up and down in aerobics classes, and so forth.

18. Lose weight. It has been estimated that shedding just ten pounds can lower blood pressure.

HERBS IN THE KITCHEN

Culinary herbs are valuable assets in the healthful kitchen. Herbs can enhance almost any meal and decrease the need for salty flavors. If a potato-and-leek chowder is tasting flat, a little dill or parsley will liven things up. When a black bean soup lacks verve, thyme and oregano will amplify the flavors. A red sauce for pasta is positively boring without basil and oregano. Salsa is plain dull without cilantro.

The world of herbs is divided into two forms, fresh and dried. Fresh leafy herbs are the leaves or shoots of plants or trees, such as basil, oregano, and parsley. When fresh herbs are dehydrated, dried herbs are born. The flavor and texture change, but the shelf life is vastly increased. Both fresh and dried herbs are indispensable tools in the high-flavor, low-sodium approach to cooking.

Some dried herbs, such as thyme and oregano, are more concentrated and earthy than their fresh counterparts. Other dried herbs, such as basil and parsley, are quite different in taste from their fresh counterparts. When substituting dried herbs for fresh herbs, the ratio is about one teaspoon of dried herbs to one tablespoon of fresh herbs.

In the best possible scenario, dried herbs should be used along with fresh herbs. Here are a few tips for cooking with herbs.

Storing Fresh Herbs: Unless you are going to use them right away, store all fresh herbs in the refrigerator. One way is to store the rinsed herbs in a plastic bag lined with a paper towel. Another way is to stand herbs bunched and upright in a vaselike container half-filled with water. Place a plastic bag around the top and chill in the refrigerator. Herbs should keep for four to five days if kept refrigerated.

Storing Dried Herbs: Store dried herbs in tightly covered containers in a cool dark place away from direct heat or sunlight (not near ovens or range tops). Dried herbs do not last on the shelf forever; after about six months the flavors become flat. Check your herb inventory the old-fashioned way—by smelling. The aroma should be crisp. Whole or crumbled herbs retain their flavor much longer than ground herbs.

Preparation Tips for Fresh Herbs: Rinse the leafy herbs briefly beneath cold running water. Drain them in a colander and shake off any excess moisture. Pat the herbs dry with a paper towel, and discard the discolored or torn leaves. Remove the remainder of the leaves by snipping or pulling them from the sprig. If cooking with an herb with a woody stem (such as thyme or rosemary), strip off the leaves from the stem.

Some dried herbs, such as thyme and oregano, are more concentrated and earthy than their fresh counterparts. Other dried herbs, such as basil and parsley, are quite different in taste from their fresh counterparts. When substituting dried herbs for fresh herbs, the ratio is about one teaspoon of dried herbs to one tablespoon of fresh herbs.

Place the herbs on a flat cutting board and chop the herbs to the desired size. If cutting chiffonade-style, stack and roll up the herbs like a cigar, then slice the roll into ribbonlike strips. Leafy herbs can also be snipped with kitchen scissors. Add the chopped herbs to the dish. If serving a hot dish, such as soup, add the herbs near the finish. If serving a cold dish (such as a vinaigrette or salad) add the herbs before refrigerating the dish and allow the herbal flavors to meld together. Generally speaking, herbs should be chopped at the last possible minute.

Preparation Tips for Dried Herbs: For maximum flavor, gently crush the leaves in a mortar and pestle (or rub the herbs between your fingers) before adding. The "bruising" will help unlock the herb's essential flavors. Unlike fresh herbs, dried herbs are best added during the cooking process.

A Cook's Guide to Culinary Herbs

All of these herbs are available in well-stocked grocery stores or farmers' markets.

Arugula is a pale green, oak-shaped leaf with a smart, peppery taste. Arugula can be used to spice up tossed gourmet salads, grain salads, tomato dishes, and vegetable soups. Also known as rocket or roquette, the Italian herb makes a spicy replacement for basil in pesto and gives salsa an interesting twist. The larger the leaf, the spicier the flavor.

Basil, the herb of pesto fame, conveys undertones of anise, mint, and black pepper. Basil is indispensable in red sauce for pasta and enlivens salad dressings, curry sauces, tomato-based soups, and skillet vegetables. Varieties include sweet basil, Thai basil, lemon basil, and opal (or purple) basil.

Chervil is a mildly flavored, anise-scented herb with a hint of parsley. Chervil can be tossed whole or chopped into leafy salads or potato dishes. To make the classic *fines herbes,* combine chervil with parsley and tarragon.

Chives are delicate, thin herbal strands that have a hint of scallion and onion. Add chives to chowders, mashed potatoes, salad dressings, and lightly flavored soups and grain dishes. Purple chive blossoms can be used as a colorful salad garnish.

Cilantro, also known as Chinese parsley or coriander, has a pungent, cleansing taste (some say it is soapy). Cilantro bears a physical resemblance to parsley. Although best known for providing the spark in salsa, cilantro can perk up a range of dishes, from gazpacho, guacamole, Indian chutney and curry dishes to spicy bean and rice salads, stir-fries, and Latin American barbecue sauces.

Dill is a light, feathery leaf with a lemony, carawaylike flavor. Dill is popular in vichyssoise, potato salad, cucumber bisque, root vegetable purées, and delicate sauces.

Mint refers to a variety of mint-scented herbs including pineapple mint, orange mint, spearmint, peppermint, and chocolate mint. Mint provides an uplifting taste to cool yogurt sauces, grain salads, berry muffins, and fruity desserts. When combined with oregano and thyme, mint adds appealing dimensions to marinades and vinaigrettes.

Oregano and *Marjoram* are fraternal twins in the herb family. The two herbs have similar appearances and flavors and can be used interchangeably. Both have a musky, pine resin fragrance and a delicate texture. Although widely used in the dried form, the fresh versions are prevalent in Mediterranean and Mexican dishes.

Parsley was chewed as a breath freshener after a meal in ancient times. The omnipresent herb can enhance almost any dish, from salad dressings, soups, and grain or bean salads to marinades, rice entrées, and pasta sauces. There are two common varieties: curly leaf (which is springy and tightly bunched) and Italian flat leaf (which is loosely bunched and slightly stronger in flavor).

Rosemary is a slender, needle-like reed with a potent pine-tree aroma; it perks up roast potatoes, Jerusalem artichokes, and flat breads such as foccacia and *bialy*. The sturdier branches of rosemary can be used as kebab skewers for grilled vegetables.

Sorrel is a large, lemon-scented leaf. Whole sorrel leaves can be tossed into a salad (like arugula) or added to soups at the last minute. Look for sorrel at farmers' markets.

Tarragon is a European herb with a distinctive aniselike flavor. It combines well with chervil, marjoram, and parsley and is a favored herb in *fines herbes,* a classic herb blend.

Thyme is an earthy herb with a pungent aroma. The oval petals enliven New England chowder, Caribbean squash bisque, barbecue marinades, vinaigrettes, and Mediterranean pasta salads. Thyme especially invigorates woodsy mushroom soups and sauces. Unlike most fresh herbs, thyme retains its flavor during the cooking process (so it can be added at any time).

Herb Blends
Some herbs are used so frequently together that their blend has a name of its own. Table 5.1 states the names of the more popular herb blends, the main herbs found in each one, and the primary uses of the blends.

SPICES IN THE KITCHEN

Where do spices come from? Spices are derived from the seeds, bark, roots, and berries harvested from tropical plants and trees. (Remember history class? Christopher Columbus was sailing in search of peppercorns and precious spices when he stumbled upon the New World.) The bounty of spices includes everything from fragrant clove buds, pungent peppercorns, and furled cinnamon bark to an abundance of ground spices. No matter how exotic, most spices are widely available and within the grasp of every cook's fingertips.

TABLE 5.1
Five Classic Herb Blends

Herb Blend	Chief Ingredients	Popular Uses
Bouquet Garni ("herb bouquet")	Whole sprigs of parsley, thyme, bay leaves, oregano, rosemary, and marjoram tied in a bunch.	Simmer the bouquet garni in soups and sauces.
Fines Herbes	Tarragon, chervil, parsley, and/or chives.	Corn chowders, stewed parsnips, fish stews, and dressings.
Herbes de Provence	Thyme, basil, savory, fennel, and lavender flowers (herbs grown in Provence).	Potato soups and salads, salad dressings, root vegetable purées.
Italian Seasonings	Oregano, basil, parsley, and thyme.	Red sauce for pasta, pizza sauce, pasta salads, sautéed vegetables.
Mediterranean Herbs	Oregano, marjoram, parsley, and thyme.	Sautéed zucchini and summer vegetables, pasta salads, vinaigrettes.

Commercially ground spices are the most common and convenient form of seasonings available. Ground spices can penetrate a dish immediately and are a great help to a cook in a hurry. Still, many cooks prefer to grind their seasonings. Whole spices such as cinnamon sticks, allspice berries, and cumin seeds offer intense flavors and piercing aromas. Whole spices and seeds are typically ground up in a spice grinder (like a coffee bean grinder) just before being added to a dish. If left whole, the spices can be wrapped in a cheesecloth (similar to a bouquet garni) and removed at the finish.

Contrary to popular opinion, spices do not last forever. Ground spices stay fresh for about six months and whole spices last up to one year. It is a good idea to periodically take an inventory of the spice rack. If a spice does not exhibit a strong aroma or robust color, it may be past its prime and ready to jettisoned. Additionally, the spice rack should be located away from direct oven heat, fans, and bright lights. Any prolonged exposure to direct heat (or steam) will cause "caking" and a loss of flavor.

Roasting Spices for a Gourmet Flavor

To further intensify the spice experience, try toasting (or roasting) whole spices. Toasting removes any moisture in the spice and extracts a deeper, more pronounced flavor. To roast, layer the whole spices or seeds on an ungreased baking pan and bake at 325 degrees F for about 10 minutes until the spices are lightly browned (stir frequently). To toast the spices in a skillet, cook over high heat for a few minutes while frequently shaking and stirring the pan. When the spices reach the smoking point, they're done. (Careful. Burnt spices have a bitter flavor.) Once toasted, the spices are ready for the spice grinder.

A Cook's Guide to Spices

Here is a guide to some of the most commonly used spices.

Allspice is a reddish brown berry grown in the tropics. (Many erroneously assume it is a mixture of "all spices.") Allspice's penetrating aroma calls up cinnamon, cloves, and nutmeg. The spice is a central flavor in Caribbean dishes such as Jamaican jerk barbecue, pumpkin bisque, West Indian curry, mango chutney, and rum cake. Allspice can replace cinnamon in banana bread, muffins, pancakes, and fruity desserts like cobbler and apple pie.

Cinnamon comes from the furled brown bark of a tropical plant. Ground cinnamon can be found in fragrant curry dishes, banana bread, pumpkin muffins, sweet breads, and fruity desserts. Cinnamon sticks can be simmered in hot beverages and rice puddings.

Cumin is a versatile spice with an earthy, musky aroma and a desert-brown hue. The spice is instrumental in Southwestern salsa, rice pilaf, black bean soup, chili, curry dishes, barbecue rubs, and marinades. Cumin goes well with coriander, oregano, red hot chilies, and other assertive seasonings.

Nutmeg and *Mace* both come from the same tropical plant. Nutmeg is a hard, nutlike seed with an oval shape, and mace is the nut's lacy outer covering. The curvy "blades of mace" are removed and ground up separately. Both nutmeg and mace add light flavors to winter squash soup, pumpkin bread, fruit cobblers, applesauce, fruit shakes, muffins, dessert salads, and, of course, piña coladas.

Paprika is unobtrusive, versatile, and colorful. The brick-red spice is actually a Hungarian pepper that has been dried and finely ground into a powder. If not for the presence of paprika, hash browns would be pallid and unexciting. A light sprinkle of paprika will perk up roasted potatoes, root vegetables, and vegetable stews and chowders.

Peppercorns refers not only to black peppercorns, but also to white, green, pink, and even red varieties. The familiar black peppercorns are really unripe green berries that have been dried and hardened. When green berries are freeze-dried, they are sold as green peppercorns. If green peppercorns are left on the vine to mature, they ripen into red berries. When red berries are soaked and dehydrated, they are transformed into white peppercorns. To further complicate matters, fancy pink peppercorns come from an entirely different plant. Ground red pepper (also called cayenne) comes from red chili peppers, not peppercorn plants.

The pungent, floral flavor of peppercorns diminishes dramatically after they are ground. One secret to creating a well-rounded, peppery sensation is to combine equal parts of white pepper and black pepper. When two or more kinds of peppers are combined, a symmetry of heat results. Blackened seasonings—a blend of several hot peppers—is a prime example of this spicing symmetry.

Red Pepper Flakes are dried and coarsely ground shards of hot red chilies. Red pepper flakes are about twice as hot as black peppercorns. Botanically speaking, red pepper flakes are not in the peppercorn family. Red pepper flakes can be used like black pepper when more heat is desired; a little goes a long way. Red pepper flakes are especially desirable in red sauces, pizza, and pasta dishes.

Turmeric is a vibrant yellowish orange spice derived from a knobby rhizome similar to ginger root. Turmeric gives table mustard its bright yellow hue. Better known for its color than its flavor, turmeric enlivens paella and risotto and invigorates almost any curry dish. A dash of turmeric brings verve to winter squash bisque and sweet potato soup. Turmeric is often called the poor man's saffron because it makes a good substitute for the world's most expensive spice.

Worldly Spice Blends

Spice blends have secured a permanent place in the world's lexicon of flavors. Mix them at home or stock up on commercial blends. (But read the labels; many contain high amounts of salt.) Table 5.2 describes the most common spice blends.

CHILI PEPPERS IN THE KITCHEN

A penchant for hot peppers is sweeping the country. From grocery stores and restaurants to farmers' markets and kitchen gardens, a bounty of colorful, curvaceous chili peppers are beckoning with culinary promises. Salsa has replaced ketchup as the most popular condiment, and bottled hot sauces are as ubiquitous as salt and pepper shakers. Chefs on the cutting edge no longer look to European cuisine for inspiration but instead explore the more adventurous hot-and-spicy fare of ethnic cultures.

Chili peppers score points in the nutrient category as well. Chilies are high in beta-carotene, vitamin C (especially red chilies), and *capsaicin*, the phytochemical that puts the "hot" in chili peppers. Fresh chilies are also low in fat and sodium. Additionally, their intense flavors make people less likely to reach for

TABLE 5.2
Six Classic Spice Blends

Spice Blend	Chief Ingredients	Popular Uses
Blackened Seasonings, also called Cajun spices	Cayenne pepper, black and white pepper, paprika, thyme, onion, garlic, and oregano	Sprinkle over grilled vegetables and fish.
Caribbean Seasonings	Nutmeg, allspice, mace, black pepper, thyme, and sometimes ground habanero peppers	Sprinkle over roasted squash, sweet potatoes, pumpkin soup, curried squash, and marinades.
Chili Powder	Red pepper, cumin, paprika, oregano, and garlic powder	Add to chili, vegetable stews, spice rubs, and bean dishes.
Chinese Five Spice	Cinnamon, star anise, cloves, ginger, and Szechwan peppercorn	Add to stir-fries, rice dishes, and soy-based sauces.
Curry Powder	Turmeric, cumin, cloves, coriander, red pepper, ginger, allspice, cinnamon, and mustard	Curry inspires spicy potato soups, vegetarian "hot pots," and fragrant stews.
Garam Masala	Cardamom, coriander, cinnamon, cumin, and cloves	Sprinkle in curry dishes, chutneys, and rice pilafs.

the salt shaker. Who needs salt, butter, or cream when you can exhilarate your taste buds with dynamic chilies?

The Allure of Chilies

The source of the chili pepper's endearing heat, *capsaicin,* has no flavor, color, or smell. The amount present in the chili determines the level of heat. (A fiery Scotch bonnet pepper contains a jackpot of capsaicin, while a sweet bell pepper has zero capsaicin.) The chemical is spread unevenly throughout the pepper but is concentrated in the membrane connecting the seeds to the cell wall.

Capsaicin coming into contact with the mouth creates the familiar burning sensation. Hot and spicy food causes our noses to run, our eyes to water, and our foreheads to form beads of sweat. Yet we go back for more. What is the allure? It seems that the presence of capsaicin triggers the brain to release endorphins, with pain-killing, pleasure-producing properties. With the next bite comes another release of endorphins. This risk-and-pleasure syndrome is similar to the thrill of riding a roller coaster. A feeling of intense fear and panic is followed rapidly by a great sense of relief—when the endorphins are deployed. With hot and spicy foods, the burn is replaced by a sense of pleasure. (Granted, I am a connoisseur of chili peppers and love fiery fare!)

A Chili Pepper Primer

From soups, salads, and sauces to pilafs, red sauces, pizza, and pasta, hot peppers enliven a variety of meals. Salsa, curries, and guacamole owe their pungent flavor to hot chilies. Chili peppers punctuate a meal with an exclamation point of flavor.

Here are a few chili pepper pointers to help you enjoy the pleasures of the piquant peppers.

Selection: Look for chilies with a smooth, taut skin and free of blemishes or wrinkles.

Preparation: To prepare a chili pepper, remove the stem and slit the pepper in half lengthwise. Slide a butter knife along the inside of the pepper, removing the seeds. (Removing the seeds tempers the heat and allows for a smoother heat distribution.) The pepper is now ready to be minced or chopped.

Protect Yourself: If you have sensitive skin, it is a good idea to wear plastic or rubber gloves when handling the peppers. Avoid touching any part of your face; any trace of hot chilies on your fingers will cause a burning sensation.

Heat Relief: If your meal is too hot, the best strategy for relief is to drink or eat a dairy product, such as milk or yogurt. Dairy products contain a protein, casein, that neutralizes the capsaicin. Drinking ice water, cola, or alcohol doesn't have much effect and may even intensify the heat.

A Cook's Guide to Chili Peppers

From mild bell peppers to incendiary habaneros, there are scores of chili peppers with varying degrees of heat and subtle flavors.

Anaheim are long, green chilies with a mild bell pepper–like flavor. Grown in California, Anaheim chilies are ideal for stuffed pepper dishes.

Cayenne peppers are long, thin chilies with a concentrated spike of intense heat. Cayenne peppers are often dried and ground into powders and hot sauces. The piquant chilies are a favorite flavor in Creole, African, and Asian dishes.

Chipotle Peppers are large jalapeño chilies that have been dried and smoked. Available canned or air packed, chipotles have a distinctive smoky nuance. (Soak the air-packed chili for 30 minutes in warm water before using.) The chilies can be substituted for bacon, pork, or dried meats in dishes with a smoky flavor.

Habaneros are one of the world's hottest pods. Brightly hued and lantern-shaped, habaneros are close relatives of Scotch bonnet peppers and display a similar scorching, blistering heat. Orange habaneros are now grown commercially in California, Texas, and the Carolinas. The chilies are prevalent in Caribbean, Yucatan, and South American cooking, especially salsas, soups, marinades, salads, and a plethora of bottled hot sauces.

Jalapeño Peppers are dark green, bullet-shaped hot chilies with a thick flesh and green pepper–like flavor. They are the most versatile chili pepper available and can spice up anything from salsas, soups, and salads to sauces, pastas, and grain dishes.

New Mexico chilies are long, tapered green or red pods that flourish in the American Southwest. The chilies produces a mellow heat and cherrylike flavor. New Mexico chilies are frequently roasted and stuffed or added to sauces, soups, and rice and bean dishes. When dried, New Mexico chilies are tied into ornamental *ristras* (holiday wreaths).

Pepperoncinis are pickled, pale green Italian peppers. Often found on salad bars, pepperoncini chilies have a fleeting, pointed heat. They are great for pasta salads, bean dishes, grain salads, and antipasto dishes.

Poblano chilies are large, forest green–purple pods with a large anvil shape and sturdy flesh. Poblanos have a raisinlike flavor and a mellow but distinctive heat that can sneak up on you. Poblanos are often roasted and stuffed or added to grain and legume dishes or hearty pots of chili. Dried poblanos are called ancho peppers.

Red Fresno chilies are similar to red jalapeños but exhibit a slightly hotter personality. Red fresnos have broad shoulders that taper to a point. The chilies are interchangeable with jalapeños and can be used in salsas, rice dishes, curries, sauces, dips, and marinades.

Rocatillo, also called *aji dulce,* has multicolored pods with a tiny patty pan squash shape. They have a sweet, citrusy flavor, bright colors, and mild heat. Rocatillos are great for salads and dips.

Scotch Bonnet Peppers have a souped-up, megawatt heat adorned with a distinctive floral flavor. Scotch bonnets come in a rainbow of colors, curvaceous shapes, and sizes. Native to Jamaica, the chilies are used in jerk barbecue, soups and stews, rice-and-peas, and a multitude of hot sauces. The name comes from its resemblance to a floppy hat worn by Scots. Scotch bonnets are also known as country pepper, Congo pepper, and Bahama mama and are interchangeable with habaneros, their close cousins.

Serrano chilies are narrow, thin pods with a prickly, fleeting heat that will catch your attention fast. Serranos can be used in salsas, soups, bean dishes, curries, and stir-fries.

Liquid Fire: Hot Sauces with Molten Flavors

The growing enthusiasm for hot-and-spicy fare has inspired a burgeoning market for bottled hot sauces. There is a vast array of hot sauces available, starting with the granddaddy of them all, Tabasco, and now including nouveau sauces made with jalapeños, Scotch bonnet peppers, habaneros, and other fiery chilies. Instead of reaching for the salt shaker, more and more people are reaching for the hot sauce.

Once you've acquired a taste for hot sauces, there will be little need for salty or buttery flavors. A few drops will perk up almost any meal, from baked potatoes, pilafs, and grains to bean salads, vegetable soups, chili, and pasta sauces. With a bottle of hot sauce present at the table, a meal will never be accused of being dull or tepid.

AROMATICS IN THE KITCHEN: GARLIC, LEMON GRASS, GINGER, AND HORSERADISH

As flavorful as herbs and spices, aromatics are essential in the flavorful diet.

Garlic

Garlic, a bulbous herb, enlivens soups, stews, stir-fries, sautés, pilafs, hummus, and pesto. Garlic brings focus to robust tomato sauces, curries, pasta salads, and bean dishes. Garlic also contains powerful antioxidants and phytochemicals, substances that lead the fight against cell damage, heart disease, and certain cancers and may even help to reduce blood cholesterol.

Each bunch of garlic contains a tight bundle of cloves wrapped in paperlike skins. To prepare fresh garlic, first remove the paper-thin skins from the cloves. (One trick is give the clove a good whack with the flat side of a knife or the palm of your hand. The impact should loosen the skins.) The cloves can be either coarsely chopped, minced, or used whole, depending on the dish.

Roasted garlic has a smoky flavor and buttery texture. To roast a head of garlic, wrap the whole bunch (unpeeled) in aluminum foil. Place the package in a preheated 350-degree F oven and bake for 40 to 45 minutes until the garlic is tender. Remove the garlic from the oven and let cool slightly before unwrapping. The skin should peel off easily, and the cloves should be soft. Add roasted garlic to soups, mashed potatoes, salads, dressings, and sauces.

Ginger Root

Ginger root is a knobby, gnarly, tan root with a clean, sharp, lemony aroma. Minced ginger can be added to curry dishes, stir-fries, salads, and soy-based dishes. Fresh ginger is a prevalent flavor in African, Asian, Caribbean, and Indian dishes.

Lemon Grass

Lemon grass is a brittle, pale green herbal stalk with a faint lemony aroma. Peel the outer sheaf and finely chop the inner core. Lemon grass can be used in stir-fries, miso-based sauces and soups, and soy-based dishes.

Horseradish

Horseradish is known for its distinctive nose-tingling sensation. Most people wouldn't recognize horseradish in its raw state, since it is primarily sold in the "prepared" form. (Fresh horseradish looks like a brown branch with an off-white flesh.) Prepared horseradish can be added to tomato sauce, dips, potato salads, mashed root vegetables, beet salads, and borscht.

SIGNATURE RECIPES FOR THE HIGH-FLAVOR, LOW-SODIUM, HEALTHY DIET

Spice Island Seasonings

Italian Seasonings

Blackened Seasonings

Jay's Salsa

Tropical Hot Sauce

Garden Herb Pesto

Spring Pasta with Mint Pesto

Spinach Pesto

Sweet Pepper–Rouille with Thyme

Jollof Vegetable Rice

Yellow Spice Rice

Lemony Artichoke Pilaf

Mexican Rice and Peas

Roasted Beet Salad

Curried Squash with Chick-Peas

Dal with Red Lentils and Sweet Potatoes

Jamaican Jerk Vegetables

Exotic Chili Stew

Curried Potatoes with Spinach

Spiced Plantains

Red Applesauce

Additional health benefits are noted with each recipe.

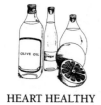

HEART HEALTHY

Spice Island Seasonings

This fragrant seasoning blend draws upon a variety of spices found on tropical islands. It is a natural ingredient to use in recipes for winter squash, plantains, curry dishes, tropical fruits, and Jamaican jerk barbecue.

1 tablespoon allspice
1 tablespoon nutmeg
$\frac{1}{2}$ tablespoon ground cloves
$\frac{1}{2}$ tablespoon cinnamon
$\frac{1}{2}$ tablespoon mace
1 teaspoon dried thyme
1 teaspoon black pepper

Combine all of the ingredients in a small mixing bowl. Spoon the seasonings into a container with a sieve top. Store in a cool, dry place.

Sprinkle the spice blend over winter squash dishes and soups, curry dishes, roasted plantains, tropical fruit chutneys and relishes, and steamed vegetables.

YIELD: ABOUT $\frac{1}{4}$ CUP

Italian Seasonings

This blend combines the herbs of the Italian kitchen. The spices will perk up any marinara, pasta salad, or tomato-based soup or stew.

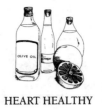

HEART HEALTHY

2 tablespoons dried parsley
2 tablespoons dried oregano
2 teaspoons dried basil
1¹/2 teaspoons black pepper
¹/2 teaspoon red pepper flakes

Combine all of the ingredients in a small mixing bowl. Spoon the seasonings into a container with a sieve-top lid. Store in a cool, dry place. Sprinkle the spice blend into red sauces for pasta, tomato-based soups and stews, ratatouille, skillet vegetable dishes, and pasta salads.

YIELD: ABOUT ¹/3 CUP

Blackened Seasonings

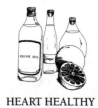

HEART HEALTHY

This famous blend of boisterous spices is easy (and cheap) to make at home. Sprinkle it over grilled vegetables, tofu, or fish—and say good-bye to the salt shaker!

2 tablespoons chili powder
1 tablespoon black pepper
2 teaspoons white pepper
2 teaspoons paprika
2 teaspoons onion powder
1 1/2 teaspoons dried thyme
1/2 teaspoon cayenne pepper

Combine all of the ingredients in a small mixing bowl. Spoon the seasonings into a container with a sieve-top lid and store in a cool, dry place.

Sprinkle the spice blend over grilled or roasted vegetables, tofu, tempeh, or grilled fish.

YIELD: ABOUT 1/3 CUP

Jay's Salsa

The best way to enjoy this salsa is to dip warm flour tortillas (not fried chips) into it. This salsa is so good you'll want to eat it for dinner.

ANTIOXIDANTS

HEART HEALTHY

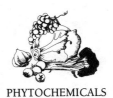

PHYTOCHEMICALS

2 ripe tomatoes, diced
1 green bell pepper, seeded and diced
1 medium yellow onion, diced
2 cloves garlic, minced
1 to 2 jalapeño peppers, seeded and minced
2 tablespoons chopped fresh cilantro
Juice of 1 lime
1 teaspoon ground cumin
1 teaspoon dried oregano
1/4 teaspoon black pepper
1/4 teaspoon salt
1/4 teaspoon cayenne pepper
1 can (16 ounces) crushed tomatoes

Combine the diced tomatoes, bell pepper, onion, garlic, jalapeño, cilantro, lime juice, cumin, oregano, pepper, salt, and cayenne in a large bowl and mix well. Place three-quarters of the mixture in a food processor fitted with a steel blade and process for 5 seconds, creating a chunky vegetable mash.

Return the mash to the bowl and add the crushed tomatoes; blend well. Chill the salsa for at least 1 hour to allow the flavors to meld together. Serve with warm flour tortillas

YIELD: 4 CUPS

HELPFUL HINT

For a salsa with more heat to it, try a different chili, such as a chipotle, serrano, or red Fresno.

Tropical Hot Sauce

ANTIOXIDANTS

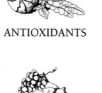

PHYTOCHEMICALS

This homemade hot sauce has a fruity heat and uplifting flavor. A little goes a long way. Almost any fresh chili can be used: serrano, jalapeño, cayenne, or if you are brave, Scotch bonnet or habanero.

4 to 6 chili peppers, seeded and chopped
1 medium carrot, peeled and diced
1$^{1}/_{2}$ cups apple cider vinegar
1 ripe mango, peeled, pitted, and diced
$^{1}/_{2}$ cup diced red onion
Juice of 1 lime
2 cloves garlic, minced
3 tablespoons brown sugar
$^{1}/_{4}$ teaspoon ground turmeric

Place all of the ingredients in a nonreactive saucepan and bring to a simmer over medium heat. Cook for 15 to 20 minutes over medium-low heat, stirring occasionally.

Remove the sauce from the heat and let cool slightly. Ladle into a food processor fitted with a steel blade or place in a blender and process for 5 seconds until smooth. Refrigerate the sauce for later use or serve immediately. The sauce should keep for several weeks in the refrigerator.

YIELD: 2 CUPS

Garden Herb Pesto

This enlightened version of pesto is fortified with tomatoes. Toss the pesto with cooked pasta or any variety of grains and beans.

ANTIOXIDANTS

4 to 6 cloves garlic
1/3 cup almonds or walnuts
2 juicy plum tomatoes, diced
1 cup packed fresh basil leaves
1 cup packed *mixture* of parsley, oregano, and mint
1/3 cup olive oil
1/2 teaspoon salt
1/2 teaspoon black pepper
1/2 cup grated Parmesan cheese

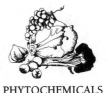

PHYTOCHEMICALS

Place the garlic and nuts in a food processor fitted with a steel blade or in a blender. Process for 5 to 10 seconds, stopping once to scrape the sides. Add the tomatoes, basil, mixed herbs, oil, salt, and pepper and process for 10 seconds more until smooth. Stop at least once to scrape the sides. Transfer the pesto to a mixing bowl and fold in the cheese. Refrigerate until ready to use.

YIELD: ABOUT 1 1/2 CUPS

Spring Pasta with Mint Pesto

ANTIOXIDANTS

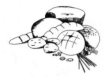

FIBER

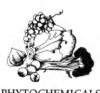

POWER EATING

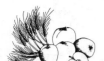

PHYTOCHEMICALS

Pasta and pesto go hand in hand. Mint lends a springlike taste to this rendition.

For the pesto:

4 large cloves garlic
1/3 cup pine nuts or diced walnuts
1 large ripe tomato, diced
1 cup packed fresh basil leaves
1 cup packed mint leaves
1/4 cup olive oil
1/2 teaspoon salt
1/2 teaspoon black pepper
1/3 to 1/2 cup grated Parmesan cheese

For the pasta:

8 ounces pasta spirals (fusilli)
1 cup cooked corn kernels
1 cup canned chick-peas, drained
1 red bell pepper, seeded and diced
8 asparagus spears, blanched
4 large scallions, chopped

To make the pesto, put the garlic and nuts in a food processor fitted with a steel blade or in a blender. Process for 5 seconds, stopping briefly to scrape the sides. Add the tomato, basil, mint, oil, salt, and pepper and process for 5 seconds more, stopping again to scrape the sides. Continue processing for 5 to 10 seconds more until smooth. Transfer to a mixing bowl and fold in the cheese. Set aside until the pasta is ready (The pesto may be made a day ahead of time and refrigerated.)

Place the pasta in enough boiling water to cover and cook for 10 to 12 minutes, occasionally stirring, until al dente. (Do not cover the pan.) Drain in a colander and cool under cold running water.

Meanwhile, in a large mixing bowl, combine the corn, chickpeas, red bell pepper, asparagus, and scallions. Fold in the pasta and pesto. Refrigerate the salad for 1 to 2 hours before serving.

Serve over a bed of leafy green lettuce.

YIELD: 4 SERVINGS

Spinach Pesto

ANTIOXIDANTS

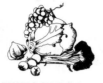

PHYTOCHEMICALS

Adding fresh spinach to a pesto recipe is an excellent way to boost the nutrient content while enhancing the flavor and presentation.

4 large cloves garlic
$1/3$ cup coarsely chopped walnuts
1 large ripe tomato, diced
1 cup packed spinach leaves
1 cup packed fresh basil leaves
$1/4$ cup olive oil
$1/2$ teaspoon salt
$1/2$ teaspoon black pepper
$1/3$ to $1/2$ cup grated Parmesan cheese

Place the garlic and nuts in a food processor fitted with a steel blade or in a blender. Process for about 5 seconds, stopping briefly to scrape the sides. Add the tomato, spinach, basil, oil, salt, and pepper and process for 5 seconds more; stop again to scrape the sides. Continue processing for 5 to 10 seconds more, until smooth. Transfer to a mixing bowl and fold in the cheese. Refrigerate the pesto until ready to use.

To enjoy the pesto: swirl into soups, spread over Italian bread, blend into pasta or potato salad, or fold into mashed potatoes.

YIELD: ABOUT $1^1/2$ CUPS

Sweet Pepper–Rouille with Thyme

Rouille is a delectable Provençal-style sauce or dip that utilizes left-over bread. This version is ideally served over pasta or rice.

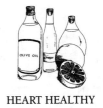

4 thick slices of French or Italian bread, crusts removed
1 1/2 cups diced roasted sweet peppers (one 12-ounce jar)
2 tablespoons olive oil
2 cloves garlic, minced
1/2 teaspoon dried thyme
1/4 teaspoon cayenne
1/4 teaspoon salt
1/2 cup lowfat milk or soy milk
1/4 cup chopped fresh parsley

In a medium mixing bowl soak the bread in warm water for about 5 seconds. Place the bread in a colander, drain, and gently squeeze out the excess water (like a sponge).

Transfer the mass of bread to a blender or food processor fitted with a steel blade. Add the sweet peppers, oil, garlic, thyme, cayenne, and salt. Process the mixture until smooth, about 5 seconds. Transfer the sauce to a medium saucepan and stir in the milk. Bring the sauce to a simmer over medium heat, stirring occasionally.

When ready, ladle the sauce over cooked pasta or rice and garnish with parsley.

YIELD: ABOUT 3 CUPS

Jollof Vegetable Rice

ANTIOXIDANTS

HEART HEALTHY

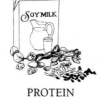

PROTEIN

POWER EATING

This festive one-pot "party dish" is rooted in West African tradition. Curry, ginger, and thyme provide an intensive combination of flavors. Greens and beans add additional nutrients and texture.

2 teaspoons canola oil
1 medium yellow onion, chopped
1 green bell pepper, seeded and diced
2 teaspoons minced ginger root
2 large tomatoes, diced
2 to 3 teaspoons curry powder
2 teaspoons dried thyme leaves
1/2 teaspoon black pepper
1/2 teaspoon salt
1 1/2 cups long grain white rice
3 cups hot water
2 cups chopped leafy greens (spinach, collards, or kale)
2 large carrots, diced
1 tablespoon tomato paste
1 can (15 ounces) black-eyed peas or red kidney beans, drained

In a large saucepan heat the oil over medium-high heat. Add the onion, bell pepper, and ginger and cook, stirring, for 5 to 7 minutes. Add the tomatoes, curry, thyme, pepper, and salt and cook, stirring, for about 2 minutes more. Stir in the rice, water, spinach, carrots, and tomato paste and bring to a boil. Cover and cook over low heat for 15 to 18 minutes until all of the liquid is absorbed.

Fluff the rice, stir in the black-eyed peas or beans, and let stand for 10 minutes before serving.

YIELD: 4 SERVINGS

HELPFUL HINT

Traditional "jollof rice" includes chopped chicken or shellfish. Either can be included (1/2 pound total) when the vegetables are sautéing.

Yellow Spice Rice

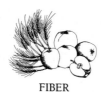

FIBER

This curry-scented rice is enriched with chick-peas and aromatic onions and garlic.

HEART HEALTHY

PROTEIN

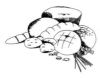

POWER EATING

1 tablespoon canola oil
1 medium red onion, diced
1 red bell pepper, seeded and diced
2 cloves garlic, minced
1 1/2 teaspoons curry powder
1 teaspoon ground cumin
1/4 teaspoon turmeric
1/2 teaspoon salt
1/2 teaspoon black pepper
1 1/2 cups long grain white rice or basmati rice
3 cups water or vegetable stock
1 can (15 ounces) chick-peas, drained
1/4 cup chopped fresh parsley

In a medium saucepan heat the oil over medium heat. Add the onion, bell pepper, and garlic and cook, stirring, for about 5 minutes. Add the curry, cumin, turmeric, salt, and pepper and cook, stirring, for 30 seconds more. Stir in the rice and water and bring to a simmer over medium-high heat. Reduce the heat to medium-low, stir in the chick-peas, and cover. Cook for 15 to 20 minutes until the rice is tender and all of the liquid is absorbed.

Remove from the heat and fluff the rice. Fold in the parsley. Let stand for 5 to 10 minutes before serving.

YIELD: 4 SERVINGS

Lemony Artichoke Pilaf

Lemon and artichokes complement each other in this enlightened pilaf.

ANTIOXIDANTS

1   tablespoon olive oil
1   medium yellow onion, diced
1   red bell pepper, seeded and diced
1   small zucchini, diced
2   cloves garlic, minced
1¹/2 cups long grain white rice
3   cups hot water
1   can (14 ounces) artichoke hearts, rinsed and
    coarsely chopped
¹/4 cup chopped fresh parsley
¹/2 teaspoon black pepper
¹/2 teaspoon salt
4   scallions, chopped
Juice of 2 lemons

HEART HEALTHY

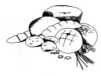

POWER EATING

In a large saucepan heat the oil over medium heat. Add the onion, bell pepper, zucchini, and garlic and cook, stirring, for about 6 minutes. Stir in rice, water, artichokes, parsley, pepper, and salt and bring to a boil. Cover and cook for 15 to 20 minutes over low heat until all of the liquid is absorbed.

Fluff the rice and blend in the scallions and lemon juice. Let stand for 5 to 10 minutes before serving.

YIELD: 4 SERVINGS

Mexican Rice and Peas

This fragrant and colorful side dish can accompany a variety of meals.

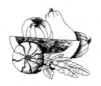

ANTIOXIDANTS

HEART HEALTHY

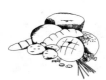

POWER EATING

1 tablespoon canola oil
1 medium yellow onion, diced
1 red bell pepper, seeded and diced
4 cloves garlic, minced
1 can (14 ounces) stewed tomatoes, drained
2 teaspoons dried oregano
1 teaspoon cumin
1/2 teaspoon turmeric
1/2 teaspoon black pepper
1/2 teaspoon salt
1 1/2 cups long grain white rice
1 cup frozen green peas
2 tablespoons chopped cilantro (optional)

In a large saucepan heat the oil over medium heat. Add the onion, bell pepper, and garlic and cook, stirring, for 5 minutes. Stir in the tomatoes, oregano, cumin, turmeric, pepper, and salt and cook for 2 minutes more. Stir in 3 cups water, the rice, and peas and bring to a simmer. Cover, reduce the heat to medium-low, and cook until all of the liquid is absorbed, about 20 minutes.

Fluff the rice, add the cilantro, and let stand for 5 to 10 minutes (still covered) before serving.

YIELD: 6 SERVINGS

Roasted Beet Salad

Beets can be roasted in the oven like a potato. Once cooked, the beets are ready to be tossed with a light herbal dressing.

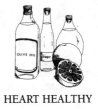

HEART HEALTHY

6 to 8 medium beets, scrubbed and rinsed
3 to 4 tablespoons canola oil
3 tablespoons red wine vinegar
2 teaspoons prepared horseradish
1 teaspoon Dijon-style mustard
1 teaspoon brown sugar
¼ cup chopped *mixture* of fresh parsley, dill, and basil
½ teaspoon ground black pepper
½ teaspoon salt

Preheat the oven to 375 degrees F.

Wrap the beets in aluminum foil and place on a baking pan. Roast for 50 minutes to 1 hour, until the beets are tender. Remove the beets from the oven, unwrap, and let cool.

Meanwhile, in a medium mixing bowl whisk together the oil, vinegar, horseradish, mustard, brown sugar, the parsley, dill, and basil mixture, pepper, and salt. When the beets are cool enough to handle, peel off any blemishes or loose skin. Coarsely chop the beets and add to the vinaigrette; coat thoroughly. Let the salad stand for 30 minutes; serve warm or chill for later.

YIELD: 4 SERVINGS

Curried Squash with Chick-Peas

The mild flavor of butternut squash is heightened with the presence of curry.

ANTIOXIDANTS

FIBER

HEART HEALTHY

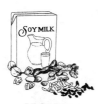

PROTEIN

2 teaspoons canola oil
1 medium red onion, diced
2 large cloves garlic, minced
1 jalapeño or other hot pepper, seeded and minced
2 ripe tomatoes, diced
2 teaspoons curry powder (preferably West Indian or Madras)
1 teaspoon ground cumin
1/2 teaspoon black pepper
1/2 teaspoon salt
1/4 teaspoon turmeric
2 1/2 to 3 cups peeled, diced butternut squash
1 can (15 ounces) chick-peas, drained

In a large saucepan heat the oil over medium-high heat. Add the onion, garlic, and jalapeño and cook, stirring, for 3 minutes. Add the tomatoes and cook, stirring, for 3 to 4 minutes more. Stir in the curry, cumin, pepper, salt, and turmeric and cook for 1 minute more.

Add the squash, 2 cups water, and chick-peas and bring to a simmer. Cook for 20 to 25 minutes over medium heat, stirring occasionally, until the squash is tender. To thicken, mash the squash against the side of the pan with the back of a spoon. Remove from the heat and let stand for 5 minutes before serving.

Serve the curry squash over rice or grains accompanied by a green vegetable.

YIELD: 4 SERVINGS

Dal with Red Lentils and Sweet Potatoes

This Indian-inspired dal can be served as a dip or a topping for potatoes or grains.

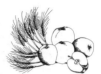

ANTIOXIDANTS

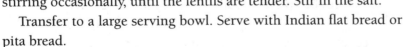

FIBER

- 2 teaspoons canola oil
- 1 medium yellow onion, finely chopped
- 2 large cloves garlic, minced
- 2 teaspoons minced fresh ginger root
- 1½ teaspoons curry powder
- 1 teaspoon ground cumin
- ¼ teaspoon ground turmeric
- ½ teaspoon black pepper
- 1 cup red lentils, rinsed
- 2 cups peeled, diced sweet potatoes
- ½ teaspoon salt
- 4 to 6 rounds of Indian flat bread (roti or nan) or pita bread

HEART HEALTHY

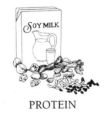

PROTEIN

In a large saucepan heat the oil over medium heat. Add the onion and garlic and cook, stirring, for 4 minutes. Stir in the ginger, curry, cumin, turmeric, and pepper and cook for 30 seconds more. Stir in the lentils and 4 cups water and bring to a simmer. Cook over medium-low heat (uncovered) for 15 minutes, stirring occasionally. Stir in the sweet potatoes and cook for 30 to 40 minutes more, stirring occasionally, until the lentils are tender. Stir in the salt.

Transfer to a large serving bowl. Serve with Indian flat bread or pita bread.

YIELD: 6 SERVINGS

HELPFUL HINT

Try serving dal with its traditional counterparts—tandoori chicken and barbecued chicken or fish.

Jamaican Jerk Vegetables

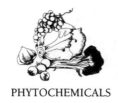

PHYTOCHEMICALS

Jamaican jerk barbecue is an earthy, pungent dish rooted in Caribbean cooking. The flavors of thyme, allspice, and chili peppers come through loud and clear.

For the marinade:

8 scallions, coarsely chopped

2 medium yellow onions, diced

$^{1}/_{2}$ Scotch bonnet or 2 large jalapeño peppers, seeded and minced

$1^{1}/_{2}$ cups low-sodium soy sauce

1 cup red wine vinegar

$^{1}/_{2}$ cup canola oil

$^{1}/_{3}$ cup brown sugar

$^{1}/_{4}$ cup chopped fresh parsley

$1^{1}/_{2}$ teaspoons dried thyme

1 teaspoon nutmeg

1 teaspoon allspice

For the vegetables:

1 pint cherry tomatoes

2 medium zucchinis, halved lengthwise and cut into $^{1}/_{2}$-inch-wide half moons

2 large yellow or green bell peppers, seeded and cut into 1-inch squares

12 ounces button mushrooms, woody stems removed

Place all of the marinade ingredients in a food processor fitted with a steel blade or in a blender. Process for 10 to 15 seconds until puréed. Transfer to a storage container and refrigerate until ready to marinate the vegetables.

Thread the vegetables onto 10-inch barbecue skewers, alternating cherry tomato, zucchini, bell pepper, mushroom, and so on. (Plan on 2 skewers per guest.) Place the skewers in 2 or more casserole dishes and pour the jerk sauce over the top. Baste the vegetables, covering them completely with the marinade. Refrigerate for 2 to 4 hours, turning the skewers after about 1 hour.

Preheat the grill until the coals are ash-gray to white.

Remove the skewers from the marinade and place on the lightly oiled grill; cook for 4 to 5 minutes on each side, or until the vegetables are tender (but not charred). Remove the finished skewers to a warm platter and grill the remaining skewers.

Serve the skewers on a bed of rice.

YIELD: 6 SERVINGS

HELPFUL HINT

Plantains make a natural accompaniment. The marinade can also be used for chicken breasts, swordfish, or shrimp.

Exotic Chili Stew

ANTIOXIDANTS

A variety of exotic dried chilies have been showing up at the market-place. Not all chilies are blistering hot, but all add invigorating flavors.

HEART HEALTHY

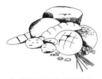

POWER EATING

2 or 3 dried New Mexico, ancho, or guajillo chilies, seeded
1 tablespoon canola oil
1 large yellow onion, diced
1 red bell pepper, seeded and diced
1 medium zucchini, diced
2 large cloves garlic, minced
1 can (14 ounces) stewed tomatoes
1 large potato, peeled and diced
1 1/2 cups corn kernels
1 tablespoon dried parsley
2 teaspoons dried oregano
1 1/2 teaspoons ground cumin
1/2 teaspoon salt
1/4 cup tomato paste

Place the chilies in an ungreased skillet. Cook over medium heat until the chilies are lightly toasted, about 2 minutes, shaking the pan and turning the chilies a few times as they cook. Remove from the heat and cover the chilies with about 1 cup simmering hot water and soak for 20 minutes. Place a lid (or plate) over the chilies to keep them from floating.

Put the chilies and about 1/2 cup soaking liquid in a blender and process until puréed, about 5 seconds. Scrape the puréed chilies into a small bowl and set aside.

In a large saucepan heat the oil over medium heat. Add the onion, bell pepper, zucchini, and garlic and cook, stirring, for 6 minutes. Stir in the puréed chilies, stewed tomatoes, 4 cups water, the potato, corn, parsley, oregano, cumin, and salt and bring to a simmer. Cook over medium-low heat until the potatoes are tender, about 20 minutes, stirring occasionally. Stir in the tomato paste and cook for 5 minutes more.

Let the stew stand for 5 to 10 minutes before serving. Ladle into bowls and serve with warm flour tortillas.

YIELD: 8 SERVINGS

HELPFUL HINT

If desired, chunks of chicken (about $\frac{1}{2}$ pound) can be added to the pot along with the sautéed vegetables.

Curried Potatoes with Spinach

Serve this aromatic curry stew over a bowl of rice (gumbo-style).

ANTIOXIDANTS

HEART HEALTHY

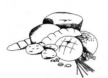

POWER EATING

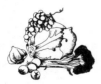

PHYTOCHEMICALS

2 to 3 teaspoons canola oil
1 medium yellow onion, diced
1 large stalk celery, sliced
2 teaspoons minced fresh ginger
1 large tomato, diced
2 teaspoons curry powder
1 teaspoon garam masala or ground coriander
1/2 teaspoon salt
1/4 teaspoon cayenne pepper
4 cups water or vegetable broth
2 1/2 cups peeled, diced potatoes
2 carrots, diced
4 cups coarsely chopped spinach
4 cups cooked rice

In a large saucepan heat the oil over medium heat. Add the onion, celery, and ginger and cook, stirring, for about 4 minutes. Add the tomato, curry powder, garam masala or coriander, salt, and cayenne and cook for 3 minutes more over low heat, stirring frequently.

Add the water or vegetable broth, potatoes, and carrots and cook for about 15 minutes over medium heat. Stir in the spinach and cook until the potatoes are tender, about 10 more minutes, stirring occasionally. Remove from the heat and let sit for 5 to 10 minutes.

Place about 1/2 cup of cooked rice into shallow bowls. Ladle the curry over the top.

YIELD: 6 SERVINGS

Spiced Plantains

Plantains, also called vegetable bananas, are popular in African, Caribbean, and Hispanic kitchens. Unlike bananas, plantains must be cooked before eating.

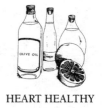

HEART HEALTHY

2 or 3 large yellow plantains
¹/₄ teaspoon nutmeg
¹/₄ teaspoon allspice or cinnamon

POWER EATING

Preheat the oven to 400 degrees F.

Cut off the tips of the plantains. Place the plantains on a baking sheet and bake for 15 to 20 minutes, until the skin is charred and puffy.

Take the plantains out of the oven and let cool for a few minutes. Slice the plantains down the center lengthwise and peel back the skin. Cut the plantains in half widthwise, sprinkle with the nutmeg and allspice or cinnamon, and place on serving plates.

YIELD: 4 SERVINGS

HELPFUL HINT

If the plantains are green and unripe, store them at room temperature for about 5 days. Storing the plantains in a paper bag can accelerate the ripening process. Despite their patchy appearance, ripe plantains are at their most desirable level—sweet and tender—when the skin is dark. This preparation is often served with Jamaican jerk chicken, fish, or vegetables.

Red Applesauce

FIBER

Homemade applesauce is a tasty way to enjoy the sweet goodness of fresh apples. Keep the skins and add a touch of spice and you'll double the pleasure.

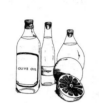

HEART HEALTHY

8 red apples, diced (do not peel)
2 tablespoons honey
$^1/_4$ teaspoon nutmeg
$^1/_4$ teaspoon allspice

Place the apples and 4 to 5 tablespoons water in a saucepan. Cook over medium heat for 25 to 30 minutes, stirring occasionally, until the apples have a mashed consistency. Stir in the honey, nutmeg, and allspice. Let the mixture cool for a few minutes.

Transfer the mashed apples to a blender and blend until smooth. (For a chunky sauce, mash the apples with a spoon by hand.) Chill for at least 1 hour before serving.

YIELD: ABOUT 4 CUPS

POWER EATING WITH COMPLEX CARBOHYDRATES: Boosting Energy with Rice, Grains, Pastas, and Potatoes

Most people think of healthful eating as an exercise in restraint. To maintain a proper diet we are implored to *reduce* the fat, *cut back* on sweets, *restrict* calories, use oils and butter *sparingly,* and desserts, well, forget about it. We eat far too much of the wrong foods and we rarely know when to stop. The prescription for our extravagant appetites and overindulging often involves moderation, caution, abstinence, and sometimes outright elimination.

Healthful eating seems to be a constant battle against the forces of temptation and dietary excess. Our mind says no, no, but our taste buds and stomach say yes, yes. Vigilance and self-control are worthy mantras, but our actions speak louder than words. Many of us could use a strong health conscience, an inner voice on a megaphone telling us to put down the candy bar *now* and no one gets hurt.

Luckily, the art of healthful eating is not entirely limited to acts of deprivation or denial. Healthy eating can be rewarding and satisfying, especially when it comes to complex carbohydrates. We are urged to eat *more* (not fewer!) complex carbohydrates and to pile our plates high with pastas, rices, grains, potatoes, and root vegetables. We can eat to our heart's content (of starches) and not feel a twinge of guilt when reaching for second helpings. The path to better health is lined with copious amounts of complex carbohydrates. The thought is positively refreshing.

Indeed, complex carbohydrates form the foundation of a healthful diet. The carbohydrate "power foods"—whole grains, brown rice, pastas, beans, yams, and fruits—provide our bodies with vital energy, stamina, and nutrients. Carbohydrate-rich foods act as high-octane fuel for our bodies while satisfying our appetites and diluting the desire to overeat. A well-balanced diet leveraged with starches might even inspire us to be more active and less sedentary and decrease the desire to yawn in the middle of the morning or afternoon. Unlike short-lived stimulants (such as coffee and chocolate), complex carbohydrates come with an enriching package of essential vitamins, minerals, and good-for-you fiber.

THE CARBOHYDRATE CONNECTION: AN IN-DEPTH LOOK

To fully appreciate the dietary merits of complex carbohydrates, it is important to understand the fundamentals of how the human body synthesizes, utilizes, and stores its energy.

There are three basic types of carbohydrates in the foods we eat: complex carbohydrates (also called starches); simple carbohydrates (also called simple sugars); and fiber, a group of indigestible substances with a bounty of health benefits. Carbohydrates are found abundantly in plant foods such as garden vegetables, potatoes, roots, legumes, brown rice, fruits, and, of course, pastas and grains. Except for the lactose present in dairy products, there are virtually no carbohydrates found in animal foods, which contain mostly protein and fat.

Starches and simple sugars are both digested by the body into glucose, a simple sugar that can be used for energy. Glucose is carried through the bloodstream and transported to the cells for use as energy. (Think of glucose as a unit of fuel, like gasoline.) Unused glucose is stored over the long term as body fat. For short-term needs, the body stores a small amount of glucose as glycogen in muscles and the liver. Glycogen is a readily available form of energy.

FROM PLANTS TO PEOPLE: HOW CARBOHYDRATES MEET OUR ENERGY NEEDS

Let's begin with a short primer on how the food we eat is converted to a life-force of energy.

Carbohydrates—such as potatoes, apples, and grains—are converted to glucose by digestive enzymes. The glucose travels in the bloodstream and is used as energy at the cellular level. Any excess glucose is stored two ways: a small amount is stored as glycogen in the muscles and liver and the majority of excess glucose is stored as body fat. When the glucose circulating in the bloodstream is depleted (i.e., low blood sugar), the body taps into the glycogen storehouses and converts the glycogen into glucose for energy.

On the other hand, when blood sugar levels are high, the pancreas releases a chemical called insulin to neutralize the glucose. Strenuous exercise can deplete both the glucose in the bloodstream and the short-term storage of glycogen. At this point the body begins to burn the warehouse of stored body fat. (Excess dietary fat and carbohydrates are stored as body fat.)

But not all carbohydrates are created equal. Potatoes and candy bars are both members of the carbohydrate family, but there are vast differences in their individual nutrient content and dietary "worthiness." Like the diverse group of dietary fats, there are both "good" and "bad" carbohydrates to be reckoned with (see Table 6.1).

Complex Carbohydrates

Complex carbohydrates, the primary constituent in starchy foods, are the good guys. In scientific jargon, complex carbohydrates are made of long chains of glucose units; some starches contain up to 1,000 units of glucose. Subsequently, our digestive enzymes take a long time to break down starches into glucose, the desired end product. As a result, glucose is gradually and slowly released into our bloodstream. This gradual digestion, absorption, and release of glucose leads to a more stable blood sugar level (a good thing). Ultimately, when eating a carbohydrate-rich diet our bodies experience a steady, long-lasting flow of energy. Eating starchy foods is akin to filling up your car with premium, clean-burning gas instead of cheap gas.

Where do complex carbohydrates come from? Plant foods, of course. It turns out that plants store carbohydrates as a form of energy as well, mostly in their seeds, roots, tubers, and stems. When we eat starchy foods, we consume this "stored" form of potent energy. It makes sense: grains such as wheat, barley, quinoa, and wild rice come from hulled seeds or kernels—small packages of energy for the next generation of plants. Tubers such as potatoes are plant storehouses of carbohydrates, as are root vegetables such as turnips and yams. Italian pastas are made from a variety of wheat called semolina; Asian noodles are made from rice, wheat, or mung beans (cellophane noodles).

Starchy foods rich in complex carbohydrates take longer to digest than most foods and tend to depress the desire to overeat or binge. This dulling of the appetite is a welcome feeling for perpetual dieters. In addition, starchy foods tend to be rich in fiber, the indigestible carbohydrate with a long résumé of health attributes.

As an added benefit, complex carbohydrates and fiber combine to slow down the absorption of glucose into the bloodstream and prevent a rapid increase (and decrease) of blood sugar levels and ease the job of the pancreas. Fiber also contributes to a sated feeling after a meal. (For more information about fiber, turn to Pillar 2: Discover the Goodness of Fiber.)

Foods rich in complex carbohydrates are also known as "mood foods." A diet low in complex carbohydrates often leads to poor concentration, fatigue, slow reflexes, bad moods, and low energy. Why? One theory holds that complex carbohydrates facilitate the production of serotonin, a chemical that relieves anxiety and depression. Serotonin is synthesized in the body from tryptophan, an amino acid found in protein. Carbohydrates seem to facilitate the body's absorption of tryptophan, which is then converted into serotonin, our natural relaxer.

As a bonus, starchy power foods often come with an entourage of beneficial components such as antioxidants and phytochemicals and tend to be low in fat. (Plant foods contain no cholesterol.) Compare this to the typical high-protein, animal-based diet, which lacks not only carbohydrates but many of these disease-fighting substances. The lack of energy-supplying complex carbohydrates may also explain why one feels sluggish after eating a large meat-based meal like roast turkey or beef. The body has to work harder to convert protein or fat into energy.

As a bonus, starchy power foods often come with an entourage of beneficial components such as antioxidants and phytochemicals and tend to be low in fat.

Simple Carbohydrates

Simple carbohydrates, commonly known as simple sugars, show up in honey, maple syrup, molasses, corn syrup, glucose, fructose, and of course, the ubiquitous table sugar, also known as sucrose. Simple carbohydrates exist naturally in fruits and vegetables. In scientific terms, as most fruits ripen, their starches are converted to simple sugars.(Bananas, kiwi fruits, mangoes, peaches, and plantains taste sweeter as they ripen.) In vegetables, the opposite reaction occurs: sweet sugars are converted to starches. (Sweet corn picked later in the season tastes starchier than corn on the cob harvested earlier in the summer.)

There is no shortage of sugar in the nation's food supply. Commercial food processors discovered a long time ago that adding simple sugars to food was a cheap and easy way to enhance the flavor. Simple sugars are a major ingredient in candy bars, soft drinks, ice cream, baked goods, desserts, and a brigade of sweetened cereals. Sugar also appears in such unlikely places as tomato sauce, canned beans, salad dressings, breads, soups, and so-called "fruit juices." Read the labels of processed foods and you'll be amazed at the breadth of products latently sweetened with simple sugars.

There is often more than one type of simple sugar listed on the same label, such as corn syrup, fructose, and maltose. Multiple listings of sweeteners can be misleading if you are attempting to keep track of the proportion of simple sugars added to the food product. For example, a salad dressing or cereal may list maltodextrin, dextrose, corn syrup, and fructose—all sugars! Add them up and simple sugars may be the number-one ingredient in that product.

What are the problems with simple sugars? Sugary foods require little digestion, go straight to the bloodstream as glucose, and contribute few health benefits. (Actually, there are no nutrients in sugar.) The body experiences a quick surge of energy, but the burst fades just as quickly. Sugary foods provide a "sugar high" but lack the long-lasting energy supplied by complex carbohydrates. A candy bar delivers a quick jolt as blood sugar levels rise, but just as quickly a "crash" follows as blood sugar levels recede. The candy bar commercials may persuade us to reach for a chocolate bar when we are feeling lethargic, but the energy boost is short-lived.

There's more bad news: processed foods high in simple sugars tend to be loaded with calories and fat and lacking in fiber (fruits are the exceptions). Processed foods also lack many of the health-enhancing nutrients found in wholesome foods. Sugar-laden junk foods deliver quick-burning calories but little long-term fuel. Sugary foods are energy-zappers, not providers.

All simple carbohydrates should not be avoided, however. Fresh fruits contain fructose but also contribute plenty of dietary fiber, antioxidants, and phytochemicals to your diet. In fact, when you have a craving for something sweet, reaching for a tasty kiwi, apple, pear, banana, or peach is an emmensely better choice than a candy bar.

COMPLEX CARBOHYDRATES ARE NOT FATTENING

Every few years a faddish diet comes along blaming complex carbohydrates for the country's "battle of the bulge." Truthfully speaking, starchy foods themselves are not overtly fattening. A baked potato, for example, has nearly zero fat. Rice is very low in fat. Once the potato or rice is on the plate, however, another story unfolds. Spreading gobs of sour cream over a baked potato or butter over rice sends the caloric meter sky high. The same story line holds for pasta. The *pasta* used in fettuccine Alfredo isn't fattening; it's the rich sauce made with artery-clogging heavy cream, butter, eggs, and cheese.

Diets that eschew starchy carbohydrates can actually do more harm than good. Carbohydrates are the most efficient source of fuel available, and when you avoid starchy foods and vegetables, you lose the whole package—fiber, vitamins, and antioxidants. The public needs to *increase* foods rich in complex carbohydrates and fiber and *decrease* the villains of the healthy diet: saturated fat, dietary cholesterol, animal protein, and sodium.

WHERE TO FIND COMPLEX CARBOHYDRATES

It is easy to include a variety of starchy power foods in a well-balanced diet. Start with the versatile potato. There are myriad

'Tis a noble goal to eat more starchy foods and cut back on sweets, but some things are easier said than done. However, no one is preaching complete abstinence from sugar, just moderation. (Life is too short to avoid dessert altogether.) The goal is to move starches (and vegetables) from the sidelines to the headlines, from the side dish to the main dish.

ways to include potatoes in salads, soups, chowders, and stews. By themselves, potatoes can be baked, shredded, boiled, or mashed. Remember to include sweet potatoes in the rotation as well.

Whole grains and rices form the infrastructure of the high-energy diet. Brown rice, quinoa, couscous, barley, wild rice, and bulgur are easy and rewarding starches to prepare. Whole grains and rices inspire a delicious range of pilafs, stir-fries, salads, soups, and hearty one-pot dishes. It is a good idea to stock your pantry with a variety of these grains and rices.

Pasta needs no introduction; it is booming in popularity. There are noodles of every shape and size, from thin strands of capellini and rice vermicelli to wide noodles of fettuccine and lo mein to squiggly corkscrews, butterfly-like bow ties (*farfalle*), wagon wheels, and old-fashioned (but lovable) elbow macaroni. Recently a new generation of whole grain pastas has captured the public's fancy. Pastas made with spelt, quinoa, buckwheat, and whole wheat are arriving at the marketplace. Gourmet pastas cook just like traditional pastas and offer additional nutrients and interesting nuances. Although they are slightly more expensive and sometimes hard to find, variety is the spice of life!

Carbohydrates contribute four calories per gram, the same as protein. Every gram of fat contains nine calories, over twice as much as carbohydrates. In addition, dietary fat is more easily converted to body fat than complex carbohydrates.

TWELVE TIPS FOR A HIGH-ENERGY DIET

Here are some ways to maintain a well-balanced, high-energy diet centered on complex carbohydrates.

1. Include brown rice and whole wheat pasta in your weekly meal plan.
2. When cooking with white rice, include cooked beans and plenty of vegetables.
3. Start your day with bran and whole grain cereals, and avoid sugar-coated brands.
4. Add fruit to your breakfast bowl (such as bananas, apples, peaches, or berries).

5. Include exotic quinoa or wild rice in salads and soups. Be adventurous.
6. Choose a baked potato over french fries, and make roasted potatoes rather than instant potato mixes.
7. Serve your baked potato with black beans, salsa, chutney, or hummus—and avoid full-fat sour cream or butter.
8. Combine pasta with tomato-based sauces, plenty of vegetables, and beans.
9. Do not add table sugar to breakfast cereals. Instead, mix in a sweetened bran cereal and fresh fruit.
10. Make starches the main dish, rather than the side dish.
11. Do not cook with nutrient-depleted instant rice or instant potatoes.
12. Do not combine pasta with heavy cream, eggs, or rich cheese sauces. Use cheese as a garnish, not as the basis for sauce.

POWER FOODS IN THE KITCHEN

Rice, grains, pasta, and potatoes are all excellent power foods and should fill the shelves of every kitchen pantry. They all have a long shelf life, are inexpensive, and are widely available.

Rice: The Amazing Grain

Rice is the world's most versatile grain. From pilaf, paella, and jambalaya to risotto, burrito, and rice pudding, there are countless enticing rice-inspired dishes. What's more, there is a "smorgasbord" of varieties to choose from. Basmati, jasmine, Wehani, wild rice, arborio, and venerable brown rice are just some of the kinds of rice available in the marketplace.

Why is rice so special? It is highly nutritious, easy to digest, economical, and a great source of complex carbohydrates. In addition, rice melds together with a wide assortment of seasonal

TABLE 6.1

The Difference Between Complex and Simple Carbohydrates

Complex Carbohydrates	Simple Carbohydrates
Good sources include starchy vegetables, brown rice, barley, grains, pastas, potatoes, sweet potatoes, and whole grain breads.	Good sources include fruits such as apples, peaches, and bananas. Also includes sweetened cereals, snacks, desserts, processed foods, and table sugar.
Breaks down slowly into glucose and provides a steady stream of efficient energy.	Goes straight to the bloodstream as glucose and burns off quickly.
Starches take longer to digest and provide a satisfied "full" feeling after a meal.	If anything, simple sugars *promote* hunger, since they are quickly burned and provide little long-term satisfaction.
Sources often contain fiber, antioxidants, and phytochemicals and are low in fat and calories.	Processed foods and sweets with added sugar are often high in dietary fat and calories as well. Sugar contains no nutritive value.
Complex carbohydrates make blood sugar levels rise and fall more smoothly and ease the job of the pancreas.	Rapid increase in blood sugar levels forces the pancreas to release insulin to neutralize the sugar.
Often contains valuable fiber, which helps prevent disease, slows absorption of glucose, and satisfies hunger.	Except for fresh fruit, sugary foods contain little or no fiber.

vegetables, pantry staples, and assertive spices. The team of rice and beans is well known, but the grain also blends with bell peppers, tomatoes, winter squash, herbs, leafy greens . . . actually, almost any vegetable. The mild grain brings a yin-and-yang harmony to more authoritative ingredients such as garlic, ginger, curry, soy, and chili peppers.

All rices are not created equal. The merits of brown rice and white rice have been compared, contrasted, and debated for years.

Brown rice is chewier, nuttier, and a better source of fiber and essential nutrients. White rice tends to be fluffier, lighter, faster cooking, and less expensive. However, white rice has been stripped of its nutrient-dense bran during the milling process. Although American rice is later enriched (with niacin, thiamin, and iron), most of the dietary fiber and other nutrients are lost.

Still, there is a place in the kitchen for exotic white rices such as arborio, basmati, jasmine, and Wild Pecan. When serving white rice it is important to include plenty of nutrient-dense ingredients in the dish. Adding beans, lentils, tofu, cruciferous vegetables, winter squash, and/or leafy greens will bring lively flavors as well as valuable nutrients to the meal. Mixing whole grains or brown rice with white rice is another way to increase the overall nutrient value while satisfying the appetite.

Here are a few general tips for preparing rice at home.

Storage: Store packages of rice in a cool, dry pantry. Unopened white rice should keep indefinitely. Brown rice has a shorter shelf life and will last for up to six months. If your brown rice is not used frequently, store it in the refrigerator.

The Difference Between Long and Short Grain: After cooking, *long grain* rices become fluffy and the grains remain separated. Long grain rices are ideal for salads and pilafs. *Short grain* rices become sticky and dense after cooking. They are good for risotto, puddings, and stuffed dishes. Both can be used in stir-fries, chili, or soups.

Preparation: Since most white rices are "enriched," they should not be rinsed before cooking—valuable nutrients will be washed down the drain. Some imported rices that are not always enriched do require rinsing. Read the label.

Risotto: For creamy risotto, an Italian rice dish, the grains are constantly stirred and absorb twice as much liquid as regular rice. Risotto is made with arborio rice, a short Italian grain. Risotto is dense and luscious, not fluffy. Grated Parmesan is swirled in at the finish.

Add a Sofrito: Healthful rice dishes (such as pilaf, biryani, and risotto) are prepared with a sofrito, an aromatic mixture of sautéed onion, garlic, peppers, mushrooms, and other vegetables. The sofrito imparts a vegetable essence to the dish while reducing the need for high-fat, high-sodium ingredients such as bouillon cubes, butter, and cream.

A GUIDE TO COOKING STOVE-TOP RICE

1. Start with a large sturdy pot with a tight-fitting lid.

2. Measure the rice and water (or broth) according to the recipe. (Usually 1 part rice to 2 parts liquid.) Combine the rice, water, and spices in the pot, stir once, and bring to a boil over medium-high heat.

3. Immediately reduce the heat to *low* and cover the pan with a tight-fitting lid. Cook for the recipe's recommended cooking time. White rice takes 15 to 20 minutes; brown rice takes 30 to 40 minutes. (Soaking brown rice ahead of time will shorten the cooking time. Remember to cook the rice in the soaking liquid.)

4. Do not stir the rice or lift the lid while it is cooking (unless you are making risotto). Stirring will cause the grains to become sticky and lumpy, not fluffy; lifting the lid will release steam and moisture.

5. Cooking times will vary slightly depending on the age and variety of rice. It is okay to peek at the rice near the finish.

6. When the rice is tender and all of the liquid is absorbed, remove the pot from the heat and fluff the grains with a fork. Let the rice stand (still covered) for 5 to 10 minutes more before serving. The rice will continue to absorb flavors while resting in the pot.

A Cook's Guide to Rice

Here is a guide to the multitude of rices that can be found in well-stocked supermarkets, natural food stores, and ethnic pantries.

Arborio is a short, pearly white grain used to make Italian risotto. Cooked arborio rice turns soft and creamy, not fluffy like most American rices. Arborio can be used in soups, rice puddings, and scores of variations of risotto. Unlike other rices, *arborio should be stirred* while it cooks.

Basmati is an aromatic, nutty rice grown in India and Pakistan. The cooked grains become slender, tender, and fluffy. (Basmati means "queen of fragrance.") Both brown basmati and white basmati are available. Another variety, *kasmati,* is a basmati-style rice grown in the United States.

Black Japonica is a blackish purple rice grown in Southeast Asia and California. Black japonica has a mild, nutty flavor and soft texture. The grain is often combined with other whole grain rices and marketed as a gourmet rice blend.

Brown Rice is a beige grain with a nutty flavor and chewy texture. Brown rice has its nutrient-dense bran layer still intact and contains twice the fiber of polished white rice. Brown rice takes about 30 to 40 minutes to cook. Varieties include short, medium, and long grains.

Jasmine Rice has a fragrant, popcorn-like aroma and nutty flavor similar to basmati. The tender grains become moist and sticky when cooked. Native to Thailand, jasmine is also called Thai Fragrant. Jasmine takes only 12 to 15 minutes to cook. A similar rice called *jasmati* is grown in the United States.

Parboiled Rice, also called "converted" rice (Uncle Ben's trademark), was invented to meet the American penchant for fluffy rice. The harvested rice is soaked in water, pressurized and steamed, and then dried. The resulting "parboiled" grains remain separate when cooked. The rice takes slightly longer to cook than regular white rice and requires slightly more liquid. (Parboiled rice should not be confused with instant rice, a product that is completely precooked and devoid of most nutrients, texture, and flavor.)

Wehani is a mahogany-colored whole grain rice marketed by Lundberg Family Farms in California. The rice has a rustic, nutty flavor and texture similar to those of brown rice. Wehani can be added to pilafs, salads, and one-pot rice dishes.

Whole Grain Rice Blends refers to a variety of gourmet rice mixtures available in the marketplace. The gourmet blends often include brown rice, wild rice, black japonica rice, and mahogany-hued rices. Whole grain rice blends are interchangeable with brown rice in most recipes. (If you haven't tried a whole grain rice blend, you're missing out!)

White Long Grain Rice is one of the most common grains in the world. To create polished white rice, the outer bran layers are removed in the milling process. In the process fiber and essential nutrients are lost. American rice is later enriched with thiamin, niacin, and riboflavin—but many of the nutrients and fiber cannot be replaced. When cooking with white rice it is important to add a variety of nutrient-dense staples to the dish such as beans, lentils, sturdy vegetables, leafy greens, squash, or tofu.

Wild Rice is not really a rice, but a dark seed of a native North American aquatic grass. The grain has a firm and chewy texture and a distinctive grassy flavor and aroma. Wild rice is harvested in the northern lakes in Minnesota and Canada (and is quite expensive). Wild rice takes about 45 to 50 minutes to cook, and 1 cup requires at least 3 cups of cooking liquid. The grain is best appreciated when blended with other whole grains.

Super Whole Grains

Super whole grains are excellent sources of complex carbohydrates, plant protein, vitamins, iron, and dietary fiber. Whole

Grains are easy to cook, but the cooking times will vary significantly depending on the variety. Couscous and bulgur cook up in minutes by steeping in hot water. Quinoa, millet, and amaranth cook as fast as white rice. Barley requires 45 minutes or longer to cook—but the wait is worth it!

1. Measure the grains and liquid according to the recipe. Combine the grains and liquid in the pot, stir it once, and bring to a simmer. Once the water is simmering, reduce the heat to low, cover, and cook for the recommended length of time.

2. Do not stir the grains while they cook (or hover over the pot!). Near the end of the cooking time it is okay to peek at the grains.

3. When the grains are tender and the liquid is completely absorbed, remove the pot from the heat and fluff the grains with a fork. Let the pot stand (still covered) for 5 to 10 minutes more before serving.

4. Grain pilafs and other one-pot grain dishes can be prepared with the help of a *sofrito,* a mixture of sautéed vegetables, herbs, and garlic. The sofrito is cooked in the pot before the grains and liquid are added. The vegetable-sofrito base will impart a delectable flavor to almost any dish of grains.

grains readily absorb other flavors in the pot and add chewy textures and substance without the fat. The family of whole grains is economical, easy to store, easy to cook, and growing in availability. To fully appreciate the goodness of super grains, stock your pantry with a wide selection.

A Cook's Guide to Super Grains

Here is a guide to the wide selection of super grains found in well-stocked supermarkets, natural food stores, and ethnic pantries.

Amaranth has beige grains shaped like poppy seeds. The ancient grains have a nutty flavor and creamy, porridgelike texture and take about 25 minutes to cook. (Amaranth also refers to the plant's leafy greens marked with streaks of red. Amaranth greens are cooked like a leafy green vegetable.)

Barley is a kernel-shaped, mild grain with "comfort food" appeal. Although most of the barley in this country is processed into malt for beer consumption, the earthy grains lend chewy substance to stews, soups, salads, and pilafs. Barley blends well with woodsy mushrooms and sturdy vegetables for an easy pilaf or wintry soup. Barley is often sold in the "pearled" form (which has been hulled or milled). It takes about 40 to 45 minutes to cook. Barley is a great source of cholesterol-lowering soluble fiber.

Bulgur refers to whole wheat berries that have been precooked, dried, cracked, and sifted. The grain is famous for inspiring tabbouleh, the Middle Eastern wheat-and-vegetable salad. To cook bulgur, simply steep the grains in boiling water for 15 to 30 minutes and drain off the excess liquid. The grains can be fluffed into multigrain salads, bean dishes, or chilled soups such as gazpacho. (Do not confuse bulgur with *cracked wheat,* a grain that has *not* been precooked and requires a slightly longer cooking time.)

Corn seems closer to a vegetable than a grain, but when it is dried and ground, cornmeal (the grain) is born. Cornmeal forms the basis of hearty accompaniments such as cornbread, polenta, corn muffins, tortillas, johnnycakes, and pancakes. Cornbread makes a savory accompaniment to spicy chili, gumbo, jambalaya, and black bean soup. Traditional cornbread tends to be rather dry, but adding corn kernels, cheese, or chipotle peppers is a way to improve the moistness and flavor.

Couscous is not technically a grain, but a tiny grainlike pasta made from fine semolina, the wheat flour used for spaghetti and other pastas. The grains take only 10 minutes to cook (by steeping in hot water). As a salad ingredient, couscous combines well with a delicate dressing such as lemon or lime vinaigrette, herbs, and legumes. For more fiber, try whole wheat couscous.

Millet is tiny beige grains with a mild, quiet flavor and has soft texture. Millet is smaller than couscous but cooks in about 25 minutes. Cooked millet makes a healthful hot cereal and is a nutritious additive to soups, salads, and pilafs. It blends well with quinoa or bulgur. Millet is high in the B vitamins, plant proteins, and minerals.

Quinoa, pronounced "keen-wa," is an ancient beige grain that has been grown in the rugged highlands of South America for centuries. The small, ringlike grains have a nutty flavor and moist, dense texture. Quinoa can be combined with (or substituted for) rice in pilafs, soups, salads, and side dishes. The versatile "mother grain" cooks in only 15 to 20 minutes—just as fast as rice. Remember to rinse uncooked quinoa thoroughly to a wash away the natural, bitter-tasting resin (saponin) that coats the grains. Quinoa is one of the best sources of plant proteins.

Spelt sounds like a fad-of-the-month grain, but, like amaranth and quinoa, it has been cultivated for centuries. Spelt is a lesser-known cousin of wheat and is processed into baking flour, cereals, and an assortment of pastas. Spelt pasta has a dark color and grainy flavor and cooks just like regular semolina pasta.

Pasta: Unlimited Pastabilities

Pasta can form the foundation of a wide gamut of healthful meals. The pasta aisles of supermarkets and natural food stores are something to marvel at. There are scores of pasta shapes, sizes, and colors. Despite the dizzying variety, traditional Italian pastas are all processed from the same durum wheat flour (also called semolina). Asian noodles (such as lo mein, rice vermicelli, and ramen noodles) are made with either rice flour, buckwheat flour, wheat flour, or, in the case of cellophane noodles, made with mung beans.

If the right routine is followed, cooking pasta can be a quick-and-easy endeavor. The goal is to serve noodles that have an "al dente" texture, meaning the texture has a slightly firm bite, not too chewy or soft and definitely not hard or mushy.

1. In a large saucepan bring plenty of water to a boil over medium-high heat (about 2½ quarts of water for every half pound of pasta). It is not necessary to add oil or salt to the boiling water.

2. Place the pasta in the boiling water, stir, and quickly return to a boil over medium-high heat. (Pasta cooked over low heat results in sticky, floury noodles.) Occasionally stir the pasta throughout the cooking process. Do not cover the pan while the pasta cooks.

3. Cook the pasta for the recommended cooking time (until al dente). It is a good idea to check for doneness one to two minutes before the allotted time has elapsed. Pull a noodle out of the water, cool it slightly, and bite into it.

4. When the pasta is ready, transfer to a colander and drain the cooking liquid. Do not run water over the pasta unless you are making a salad dish.

5. Transfer the cooked pasta to warm serving plates and serve with sauce at once. (See Table 6.2.)

In recent years there has been an avalanche of gourmet pastas. The new class of pastas can include an assortment of ingredients such as whole wheat flour, spinach, tomatoes, beets, quinoa, spelt, Jerusalem artichokes, garlic, and basil. Specialty pastas made with whole grains offer additional nutrients and alluring flavors and are worth a try.

A Cook's Guide to Gourmet Pastas

Stock your pantry with a variety of pastas and you will never get bored of this nourishing staple.

Quinoa Spaghetti, made from quinoa flour, has a nutty nuance. It cooks in minutes.

Rice Noodles are quick-cooking Asian pastas. Rice noodles are sold as thin noodles (called rice sticks or vermicelli), flat, fettuccine-like noodles, or spaghetti-shaped noodles. Rice noodles are ideal for stir-fries and soy-based salads.

Soba Noodles are long, flat Japanese noodles that resemble spaghetti. They are usually made with buckwheat flour (and also called buckwheat noodles).

Somen refers to thin, quick-cooking, Japanese white noodles. Somen noodles have a texture similar to capellini and are often served cold as a salad dish.

Spelt Spaghetti is a dark-hued pasta made with spelt flour, an ancient grain. Spelt spaghetti is interchangeable with Italian spaghetti.

Udon Noodles are flat Japanese noodles with a shape similar to linguini. Udon is made from whole wheat or rice flour and can be used in stir-fries and soups.

Whole Wheat Spaghetti is not as refined as regular spaghetti but contains more fiber. Wheat spaghetti is interchangeable with Italian spaghetti.

Plentiful Potatoes

Potatoes could be described in just one word: versatile. Potatoes can be baked, boiled, roasted, mashed, steamed, and barbecued. Potatoes inspire myriad soups, stews, and hearty one-pot dishes. Potatoes add substance and complex carbohydrates to a meal and bring a sense of balance to more assertive flavors.

The selection of potatoes has greatly expanded in recent years. The varieties include long whites, reds, sweet potatoes (not really potatoes, but roots), Yukon Golds, Russets, all-purpose, and even blue and purple potatoes. While most potatoes are

TABLE 6.2

Serving Pasta with Maximum Flavor and Minimum Fat

Pasta Do's	Pasta Don'ts
Do serve pasta with a variety of red tomato sauces.	Don't serve pasta with white sauces made with heavy cream and eggs.
Do include an array of vegetables in a pasta dish, such as broccoli, asparagus, green beans, chick-peas, leafy greens, and beets.	Don't add high-fat sausages, bacon, or fatty meatballs to pasta dishes.
Do experiment with whole grain pastas.	Don't drench pasta in a sea of butter.
Do use cheese as a garnish for pasta, not as a main ingredient.	Don't serve pasta dishes that call for cheese as a main ingredient (lasagna, manicotti, or cheese sauces).
Do order pasta with marinara sauces at restaurants.	Don't order pasta made with fatty white sauces such as fettuccine Alfredo.

interchangeable, they are grouped by their starch content: high, medium, and low.

High-starch potatoes have a "floury" flavor and fluffy texture and make the best baked potatoes. Russets, also known as baking potatoes, are the best-known variety. Idaho potatoes are synonymous with Russet baking potatoes, but Russets can be grown almost anywhere.

All-purpose, or boiling, potatoes are medium-starch potatoes. All-purpose potatoes hold up well in boiled water and can be baked, mashed, roasted, or added to soups or salads.

Low-starch potatoes have a firm texture and waxy finish. Red potatoes (also called new potatoes) and Yukon Gold are low-starch potatoes. Low-starch potatoes are great for salads and barbecuing.

Potato Pointers

Here are a few tips on preparing potatoes.

Storage: Always store potatoes in a cool, dark place. Direct sunshine or heat will hasten the demise of a good potato. Do not refrigerate them. The high-energy starches will turn to sugars. Never store potatoes in a plastic bag. Tubers need to breathe. Store potatoes either in a brown paper bag or loosely piled in a plastic bin.

Selection: Discard any potatoes covered with a potentially toxic green hue. Also, remove any sprouts and blemishes before cooking.

THE THREE-STEP METHOD TO BAKING THE PERFECT POTATO

It is easy to bake perfect potatoes.

1. Scrub the potato with a vegetable brush and pierce the skin with a fork several times. If you prefer a crunchy skin, bake the potatoes unwrapped. (Wrapping the potato in foil steams the potato and yields a soft skin.)

2. Place the potato on a baking pan and bake in a *preheated* oven set at 400 degrees F. Bake for about one hour or until the potato is easily pierced with a fork.

3. Remove the potato from the oven. To serve, slit the potato down the center, fluff up the pulp, and spoon on a healthy topping. Enjoy!

SIGNATURE RECIPES FOR THE CARBOHYDRATE-RICH, HEALTHY DIET

Wild Rice and Split Pea Soup

Wild Rice and Barley Soup

Power Chowder

Mexican Minestrone

Bulgur and Couscous Vegetable Pilaf

Orzo, Rice, and Sweet Pea Pilaf

Multigrain Vegetable Pilaf

Asparagus Pilaf with Artichokes

Powerhouse Pilaf

Farmers' Market Risotto

Asparagus and Wild Mushroom Risotto

Collard Brown Rice and Peas

Gourmet Spaghetti with Braised Greens

Wheat Spaghetti with Double Mushroom Marinara

Pasta Salad with Chick-Peas and Artichokes

Warm Millet and Corn Salad with Lime

Roasted Beet and Potato Salad

Whole Grain Salad with Beans and Corn

Smashed Potatoes with Spicy Black Beans

Sweet Pepper Polenta

Additional health benefits are noted with each recipe.

Wild Rice and Split Pea Soup

ANTIOXIDANTS

This is a satisfying tureen of grains and legumes. It is a soothing anti-dote for a cold-weather day.

1 tablespoon canola oil
1 large red onion, diced
2 stalks celery, chopped
12 ounces button mushrooms, sliced
2 or 3 large cloves garlic, minced
1 cup yellow or green split peas, rinsed
2 large carrots, diced
2 cups diced white potatoes
$^1/_2$ cup wild rice
2 tablespoons dried parsley
2 teaspoons dried oregano
1 teaspoon black pepper
1 teaspoon salt

FIBER

HEART HEALTHY

In a large saucepan heat the oil over medium-high heat. Add the onion, celery, mushrooms, and garlic and cook, stirring, for about 7 minutes. Stir in 10 cups water, the split peas, carrots, potatoes, wild rice, parsley, oregano, and pepper and bring to a simmer. Cook for 1$^1/_2$ to 2 hours over medium-low heat until the split peas are tender, stirring occasionally.

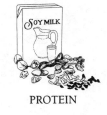

PROTEIN

Stir in the salt and cook for 5 minutes more. Remove from the heat and let stand for 5 to 10 minutes before serving. Ladle the soup into bowls and serve with whole grain bread.

YIELD: 6 SERVINGS

HELPFUL HINT

Wild rice is available in the grain section of natural food stores and well-stocked supermarkets.

Wild Rice and Barley Soup

ANTIOXIDANTS

FIBER

HEART HEALTHY

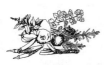

FIRE AND SPICE

This soup offers wholesome flavors and stick-to-your-ribs textures. There's also plenty of soluble fiber and starchy carbohydrates.

1 tablespoon canola oil
12 ounces button mushrooms, sliced
1 red bell pepper, seeded and diced
1 medium yellow onion, diced
2 large cloves garlic, minced
1/4 cup barley
1/4 cup wild rice
1/4 cup dry white wine
1 sweet potato, diced
2 teaspoons dried oregano
1/2 teaspoon dried thyme
1/2 teaspoon salt
1/2 teaspoon black pepper

In a large saucepan heat the oil over medium heat. Add the mushrooms, bell pepper, onion, and garlic and cook for 8 to 10 minutes, stirring frequently. Add 6 cups water, the barley, wild rice, and wine and bring to a simmer; cook for 10 minutes. Add the sweet potato, oregano, thyme, salt, and pepper and cook for 35 minutes over medium-low heat, stirring occasionally. Let the soup stand for several minutes before serving.

Ladle into bowls and serve with dark bread.

YIELD: 6 SERVINGS

Power Chowder

This chunky soup of sweet potatoes, corn, and turnips will please your palate, satisfy your appetite, and restore your energy.

ANTIOXIDANTS

1 tablespoon olive oil
1 medium yellow onion, diced
1 green bell pepper, seeded and diced
2 stalks celery, chopped
3 or 4 cloves garlic, minced
6 cups water or vegetable broth
2 medium turnips, peeled and diced
1 large sweet potato, diced
2 teaspoons dried oregano
$1/2$ teaspoon salt
$1/2$ teaspoon black pepper
1 can (15 ounces) white kidney beans, drained
1 can (14 ounces) corn kernels, drained

FIBER

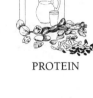

PROTEIN

In a large saucepan heat the oil over medium heat. Add the onion, bell pepper, celery, and garlic and cook, stirring, for about 6 minutes. Add the water, turnips, sweet potato, oregano, salt, and pepper and bring to a simmer. Cook for 20 minutes over medium heat, stirring occasionally. Stir in the beans and corn and cook for 10 minutes more.

PHYTOCHEMICALS

Remove from the heat and let stand for 10 minutes before serving. To thicken, mash the potatoes against the side of the pan with the back of a spoon.

Ladle the soup into bowls and serve with warm bread.

YIELD: 6 SERVINGS

Mexican Minestrone

This vegetable and noodle soup makes a light lunch or hearty appetizer. The combination of herbs and chili peppers provides a zip of spicy flavor.

ANTIOXIDANTS

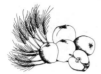

FIBER

PROTEIN

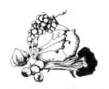

PHYTOCHEMICALS

1   tablespoon canola oil
2   large carrots, diced
1   medium yellow onion, diced
1   red or green bell pepper, seeded and diced
2 or 3 cloves garlic, minced
1   jalapeño or serrano chili, seeded and minced
2   cans (14½ ounces each) vegetable broth
2   tablespoons tomato paste
2   teaspoons dried oregano
1   teaspoon ground cumin
½   teaspoon black pepper
4   ounces spaghetti or linguini, snapped in half
1   cup cooked red kidney beans
1   cup corn kernels
2   tablespoons chopped fresh cilantro (optional)

In a large saucepan heat the oil over medium-high heat. Add the carrots, onion, bell pepper, garlic, and chili pepper and cook for 7 minutes, stirring frequently. Add the broth, tomato paste, oregano, cumin, and pepper and bring to a simmer over medium-high heat, stirring occasionally. Stir in the pasta, beans, and corn and return to a simmer. Cook, stirring occasionally, for 8 to 12 minutes over medium-high heat until the pasta is al dente. Remove from the heat and stir in the cilantro. Let stand for a few minutes before serving.

Ladle into shallow bowls and serve with flour tortillas.

YIELD: 4 SERVINGS

HELPFUL HINT

For a flavorful variation, try a gourmet spaghetti such as corn, quinoa, or whole wheat pasta. Chicken stock may be used in place of the vegetable broth.

Bulgur and Couscous Vegetable Pilaf

FIBER

HEART HEALTHY

Combining grains in one pot is an easy way to enjoy well-rounded flavors and complementary nutrients. Quick-cooking bulgur and couscous make a natural pair.

1 tablespoon canola oil
1 medium yellow onion, diced
1 bell pepper, seeded and diced
1 small zucchini, diced
10 to 12 button mushrooms, sliced
2 large cloves garlic, minced
2 teaspoons curry powder
$^{1}/_{2}$ teaspoon salt
$^{1}/_{2}$ teaspoon black pepper
1 cup couscous (preferably whole wheat)
1 cup bulgur
1 can (15 ounces) chick-peas, drained

In a medium saucepan heat the oil over medium-high heat. Add the onion, bell pepper, zucchini, mushrooms, and garlic and cook, stirring, for 5 to 7 minutes. Stir in $3^{1}/_{2}$ cups water, the curry, salt, and pepper and bring to a simmer. Stir in the couscous, bulgur, and chick-peas and cover the pan. Remove from the heat and let stand for about 15 minutes.

Fluff the grains and serve at once.

YIELD: 4 SERVINGS

Orzo, Rice, and Sweet Pea Pilaf

Orzo, a pasta with an elliptical shape, blends well with rice in a variety of pilafs and one-pot dishes.

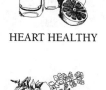

HEART HEALTHY

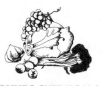

FIRE AND SPICE

PHYTOCHEMICALS

- 1 tablespoon olive oil
- 1 medium yellow onion, chopped
- 2 or 3 cloves garlic, minced
- 1 cup long grain white rice
- 1/2 cup orzo
- 1/2 teaspoon salt
- 1/2 teaspoon black pepper
- 1/4 teaspoon turmeric
- 1 cup green peas, fresh or frozen
- 1/4 cup chopped pimientos (optional)
- 2 tablespoons chopped fresh parsley

In a medium saucepan heat the oil over medium heat. Add the onion and garlic and cook, stirring, for 4 minutes. Stir in the rice, orzo, salt, pepper, and turmeric and cook for 1 minute more over low heat, stirring frequently. Add 2³/4 cups water, the green peas, and pimientos and bring to a simmer. Cover and cook for 15 to 20 minutes over low heat.

Remove from the heat, fluff the grains, and blend in the parsley. Let stand for 5 to 10 minutes (covered) before serving.

YIELD: 4 SERVINGS

HELPFUL HINT

Orzo, also called rosa maria, is available in the pasta section of grocery stores.

Multigrain Vegetable Pilaf

ANTIOXIDANTS

HEART HEALTHY

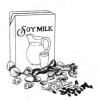

PROTEIN

This savory dish is picturesque as well as healthful. A trio of grains form a delectable alliance.

1   tablespoon canola oil
8 to 10 button mushrooms, chopped
2   carrots, diced
1   medium yellow onion, chopped
1   green or red bell pepper, seeded and diced
2 or 3 cloves garlic, minced
3   cups vegetable broth or water
1   cup brown rice or brown basmati rice
1/4 cup wild rice
1   teaspoon curry powder
1/2 teaspoon black pepper
1/2 teaspoon salt
1/2 cup couscous (whole wheat or regular)
1/2 cup boiling water

In a large saucepan heat the oil over medium heat. Add the mushrooms, carrots, onion, bell pepper, and garlic and cook, stirring, for 6 to 7 minutes. Add the broth or water, both rices, curry, pepper, and salt, stir, and bring to a boil over medium-high heat. Cover and cook over low heat for 40 to 45 minutes until the grains are tender.

Meanwhile, in a small saucepan or bowl combine the couscous and boiling water. Cover and set aside for at least 15 minutes.

When the pilaf is done, fluff the grains and fold in the couscous. Let stand for 5 to 10 minutes before serving.

YIELD: 4 SERVINGS

Asparagus Pilaf with Artichokes

Two regal vegetables, asparagus and artichokes, combine with rice for a nourishing pilaf.

1 tablespoon canola oil
1 medium yellow onion, diced
8 to 10 button mushrooms, chopped
2 large cloves garlic, minced
1¹/₂ cups long grain white rice
3¹/₂ cups water or vegetable broth
1 can (14 ounces) artichoke hearts, rinsed and
    coarsely chopped
10 to 12 asparagus spears, trimmed and cut into 1-inch pieces
¹/₄ cup chopped fresh parsley
1 teaspoon curry powder
¹/₂ teaspoon black pepper
¹/₂ teaspoon salt
Juice of 1 or 2 lemons (optional)

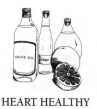

HEART HEALTHY

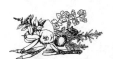

FIRE AND SPICE

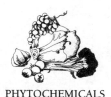

PHYTOCHEMICALS

In a medium saucepan heat the oil over high heat. Add the onion, mushrooms, and garlic and cook, stirring, for about 5 minutes. Stir in the rice, water or broth, artichokes, asparagus, parsley, curry, pepper, and salt and bring to a boil. Cover and cook for 17 to 20 minutes over low heat until the rice is tender.

Fluff the rice and let stand for 5 to 10 minutes before serving. If desired, squeeze the lemon juice over the pilaf.

YIELD: 4 SERVINGS

Powerhouse Pilaf

FIBER

This hearty one-pot dish of barley, wild rice, and lentils is packed with comfortable flavors and soothing textures. A hint of curry provides a nice yellow hue.

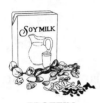

HEART HEALTHY

PROTEIN

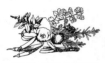

FIRE AND SPICE

1 tablespoon canola oil
1 medium yellow onion, diced
1 red bell pepper, seeded and diced
8 ounces button mushrooms, chopped
3 or 4 cloves garlic, minced
1½ teaspoons curry powder
½ cup pearl barley
¼ cup wild rice
¼ cup lentils
½ teaspoon black pepper
½ teaspoon salt

In a medium saucepan heat the oil over high heat. Add the onion, bell pepper, mushrooms, and garlic and cook, stirring, for about 6 minutes. Stir in the curry powder and cook, stirring, for 1 minute more. Stir in 4 cups water, the barley, wild rice, lentils, pepper, and salt and bring to a boil. Cover and cook over medium-low heat until all of the liquid is absorbed, about 40 to 45 minutes. Stir the grains every 10 minutes or so.

Fluff the grains and let stand for 5 to 10 minutes before serving.

YIELD: 4 SERVINGS

Farmers' Market Risotto

This velvety dish of creamy grains and summer vegetables offers a cornucopia of nourishing flavors.

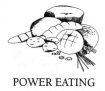

POWER EATING

2 tablespoons olive oil
2 medium yellow onions, chopped
12 ounces button mushrooms, sliced
1 red bell pepper, diced
4 cloves garlic, minced
2 cups arborio rice
1/2 cup dry white wine
1 teaspoon white pepper
1 teaspoon salt
3/4 teaspoon ground turmeric
4 ounces green beans, chopped
1/2 cup chopped fresh parsley
1/2 cup grated Parmesan or Romano cheese

In a large saucepan heat the oil over medium-high heat. Add the onion, mushrooms, bell pepper, and garlic. Cook, stirring, for about 7 minutes. Add the rice, 3 cups water, the wine, pepper, salt, and turmeric. Cook (uncovered) over medium-low heat for about 10 minutes, stirring frequently.

Stir in 2 1/2 cups water, the green beans, and parsley. Cook for 12 to 15 minutes more, continuing to stir, until the rice is tender.

Remove from the heat and stir in the cheese. Let stand for a few minutes before serving. Serve with warm Italian bread.

YIELD: 6 SERVINGS

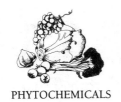

Asparagus and Wild Mushroom Risotto

PHYTOCHEMICALS

If there was a hall of fame for dishes, this risotto would be a charter member.

1 tablespoon olive oil
1 medium yellow onion, chopped
4 ounces oyster mushrooms, sliced
10 to 12 button mushrooms, sliced
1 medium portobello mushroom, sliced
2 cloves garlic, minced
1½ cups arborio rice
4½ cups hot water
½ cup dry white wine
½ teaspoon white pepper
½ teaspoon salt
½ teaspoon turmeric
10 to 12 asparagus spears, trimmed and cut into 1-inch sections
2 tablespoons chopped fresh parsley
⅓ cup grated Romano cheese

In a large saucepan heat the oil over medium heat. Add the onion, mushrooms, and garlic and cook, stirring, for about 5 to 6 minutes. Add the rice, 2 cups hot water, wine, pepper, salt, and turmeric. Cook (uncovered) over medium-low heat for about 10 minutes, stirring frequently.

Stir in the remaining 2½ cups water, asparagus, and parsley. Cook for about 12 minutes more, continuing to stir, until the rice is tender.

Remove from the heat and stir in the cheese. Let stand for a few minutes before serving. Serve with warm Italian bread.

YIELD: 4 SERVINGS

HELPFUL HINT

For a seafood risotto, add about a dozen shrimp along with the rice and cook the risotto with chicken stock.

Collard Brown Rice and Peas

ANTIOXIDANTS

This one-pot dish combines nourishing brown rice with antioxidant-rich collard greens and carrots. Other greens such as kale or chard can also be used.

FIBER

1 tablespoon canola oil
1 medium yellow onion, diced
2 cloves garlic, minced
4 cups packed collard greens (cut chiffonade-style)
3 cups water or vegetable broth
1¼ cups long grain brown rice
1 large carrot, diced
½ teaspoon salt
½ teaspoon black pepper
1 cup cooked black-eyed peas
¼ cup chopped fresh parsley

PROTEIN

In a medium saucepan heat the oil over medium-high heat. Add the onion and garlic and cook, stirring, for about 4 minutes. Stir in the collard greens and cook, stirring, for about 1 minute more. Add the water, rice, carrot, salt, and pepper and bring to a boil. Cover and cook for 30 to 35 minutes over medium-low heat. Fold in the black-eyed peas and parsley and turn off the heat. Let stand for 5 to 10 minutes before serving.

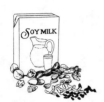

PHYTOCHEMICALS

YIELD: 4 SERVINGS

HELPFUL HINT

"Chiffonade" means cutting the greens into ribbonlike strips. Simply roll the collard greens into a cigar shape and thinly slice crosswise at an angle.

Gourmet Spaghetti with Braised Greens

This dish highlights one of the many whole grain pastas coming to a marketplace near you.

ANTIOXIDANTS

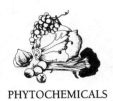

PHYTOCHEMICALS

1 tablespoon canola oil
2 or 3 cloves garlic, minced
1 bunch green or red chard (about 1 pound), trimmed and cut into strips
$1/4$ cup vegetable broth or water
$1/2$ teaspoon black pepper
$1/2$ teaspoon salt
8 ounces whole wheat spaghetti or spelt spaghetti
$1/4$ cup grated Parmesan or Romano cheese

In a large, wide skillet heat the oil over medium heat. Add the garlic and cook, stirring, for 2 minutes. Stir in the chard, broth, pepper, and salt. Cook for 4 to 5 minutes, stirring frequently, until the greens are wilted.

Meanwhile, in a large saucepan bring 3 quarts of water to a boil over medium-high heat. Place the spaghetti in the boiling water, stir, and return to a boil. Cook for about 6 to 8 minutes, until al dente, stirring occasionally. Drain in a colander.

Using tongs transfer the pasta to a large serving bowl. Add the cooked chard and toss together. Lightly sprinkle the Parmesan cheese over the top. Serve at once.

YIELD: 4 SERVINGS

Wheat Spaghetti with Double Mushroom Marinara

ANTIOXIDANTS

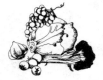

PHYTOCHEMICALS

Whole grain noodles are embellished with lycopene-rich tomatoes and woodsy mushrooms.

2 tablespoons dry red wine

1 tablespoon olive oil

12 ounces button mushrooms, sliced

4 ounces wild mushrooms (such as oyster, crimini, or shiitake), sliced

1 small yellow onion, chopped

2 or 3 cloves garlic, minced

1 can (14 ounces) stewed tomatoes

1 can (14 ounces) tomato purée

2 teaspoons dried oregano

1 teaspoon dried basil

$^1/_2$ teaspoon red pepper flakes

$^1/_2$ teaspoon salt

8 ounces whole wheat or regular spaghetti

$^1/_4$ cup grated Parmesan cheese (optional)

In a large saucepan heat the wine and oil over medium heat. Add the mushrooms, onion, and garlic and cook, stirring, for 7 to 9 minutes. Stir in the stewed tomatoes, tomato purée, oregano, basil, red pepper flakes, and salt. Reduce the heat to low and simmer for 15 to 20 minutes, stirring occasionally. (Partially cover the pan if the sauce splatters.)

Meanwhile, in another large saucepan bring 3 quarts of water to a boil over medium-high heat. Place the pasta in the boiling water, stir, and return to a boil. Cook for 8 to 10 minutes, until al dente, stirring occasionally. Drain in a colander.

When the sauce is ready, transfer the spaghetti to warm serving plates and spoon the sauce over the top. If desired, sprinkle with Parmesan cheese.

YIELD: 4 SERVINGS

HELPFUL HINT

Add a few leaves of chopped fresh arugula or basil to the sauce near the finish.

Pasta Salad with Chick-Peas and Artichokes

FIBER

HEART HEALTHY

PROTEIN

An herb-scented vinaigrette enhances this light salad of pasta, artichokes, and beans.

8 ounces rotini pasta (spirals)
1 can (15 ounces) chick-peas, drained
1 can (14 ounces) artichoke hearts, rinsed and drained
4 whole scallions, chopped
2 tomatoes, diced
2 large cloves garlic, minced
3 tablespoons balsamic or red wine vinegar
2 tablespoons canola oil
1/4 cup chopped fresh parsley
2 teaspoons dried oregano
1/2 teaspoon black pepper
1/2 teaspoon salt
1/4 cup grated Parmesan cheese

In a large saucepan bring 3 quarts of water to a boil over medium-high heat. Place the pasta in the boiling water, stir, and return to a boil. Cook until al dente, 8 to 10 minutes, stirring occasionally. Drain in a colander and cool under cold running water.

Meanwhile, in a large mixing bowl combine the remaining ingredients and toss together. Blend in the cooked pasta. Chill the salad for 1 to 2 hours to allow the flavors to meld together.

YIELD: 6 SERVINGS

Warm Millet and Corn Salad with Lime

Millet has a texture similar to couscous. For this salad it is complemented with lime, herbs, and confetti vegetables.

FIBER

1 cup millet
4 scallions, chopped
1¹/₂ cups cooked corn kernels
1 cup cooked chick-peas or black beans
1 large tomato, diced
2 cloves garlic, minced
2 tablespoons chopped fresh herbs (such as cilantro or basil)
1 tablespoon canola or olive oil
¹/₂ teaspoon salt
¹/₂ teaspoon black pepper
Juice of 1 lime

HEART HEALTHY

PROTEIN

In a medium saucepan combine the millet and 1¹/₂ cups water and bring to a simmer over medium-high heat. Cover loosely and cook for 20 to 25 minutes until all of the liquid is absorbed. Fluff the grains and set aside for 5 minutes (still covered).

Meanwhile, in a medium mixing bowl, combine the remaining ingredients and toss together thoroughly. Blend in the cooked millet grains. Serve the salad at once or chill for later.

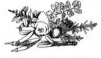

FIRE AND SPICE

YIELD: 4 SERVINGS

Roasted Beet and Potato Salad

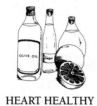

HEART HEALTHY

The venerable potato salad is reinvigorated with the addition of magenta-hued beets and vibrant herbs. Sunflower seeds add a nice crunchiness.

4 or 5 medium beets, scrubbed
2 cups diced Yukon Gold or new red potatoes
2 tablespoons canola oil
2 tablespoons apple cider vinegar
1 tablespoon prepared horseradish
1 tablespoon Dijon-style mustard
$1/4$ cup chopped fresh dill or parsley
$1/2$ teaspoon black pepper
$1/2$ teaspoon salt
2 stalks celery, diced
1 medium red onion, finely chopped
3 or 4 tablespoons sunflower seeds (optional)

Preheat the oven to 400 degrees F.

Wrap the beets in aluminum foil and place on a baking pan. Roast for 50 minutes to 1 hour until the beets are tender. Remove the beets from the oven, unwrap, and let cool. Slip off the skins and coarsely chop the beets.

Meanwhile, in a saucepan place the potatoes in boiling water to cover. Cook for about 15 minutes over medium-high heat until tender. Drain and cool under cold running water.

In a mixing bowl whisk together the oil, vinegar, horseradish, mustard, dill or parsley, pepper, and salt. Add the beets, potatoes, celery, onion, and seeds and blend together. Chill for at least 1 hour before serving. Serve over a bed of leaf lettuce.

YIELD: 4 SERVINGS

HELPFUL HINT

Other leafy herbs such as arugula, watercress, and tarragon can also be added to the salad.

Whole Grain Salad
with Beans and Corn

FIBER

HEART HEALTHY

PROTEIN

Herbs and fresh lime give this earthy salad a tangy lift, while beans and whole grains provide the substance. There is a growing variety of whole grain "gourmet" rice blends to choose from at well-stocked grocery stores.

1 cup whole grain rice blend
1 can (15 ounces) black beans or small red beans, drained
1 can (11 ounces) corn kernels, drained
2 tomatoes, diced
1 cucumber, diced (peeled if waxed)
1 tablespoon canola oil
Juice of 1 to 2 lemons
$^1/_4$ cup chopped fresh parsley
2 teaspoons dried oregano
$^1/_2$ teaspoon black pepper
$^1/_2$ teaspoon salt

In a medium saucepan combine the rice blend and $2^1/_2$ cups water and bring to a boil over medium-high heat. Reduce the heat to low, cover, and cook until all of the liquid is absorbed, about 30 minutes. Remove from the heat and fluff the rice. Let stand for 5 to 10 minutes.

Meanwhile, in a large mixing bowl combine the remaining ingredients and toss together thoroughly. Blend in the warm rice. Chill the salad for 2 hours to allow the flavors to meld together.

YIELD: 6 SERVINGS

Smashed Potatoes with
Spicy Black Beans

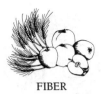

FIBER

Black beans make a healthful topping for baked potatoes—and are far healthier than sour cream or butter.

HEART HEALTHY

4 Russet baking potatoes
1 can (15 ounces) black beans or red kidney beans
1 tablespoon canola oil
1 small red onion, diced
1 large tomato, diced
1 jalapeño or other chili pepper, seeded and minced (optional)
1 teaspoon ground cumin
1/2 teaspoon black pepper
2 tablespoons chopped fresh cilantro

PROTEIN

Preheat the oven to 400 degrees F.

Scrub the potatoes and pierce the skin with a fork several times. Place the potatoes on a baking pan and bake for about one hour, until tender.

Meanwhile, drain the beans, reserving 1/4 cup of the liquid. In a medium saucepan heat the oil over medium heat. Add the onion, tomato, and jalapeño (if desired). Cook, stirring, for about 4 minutes. Stir in the beans, liquid, cumin, and pepper and cook for about 4 minutes more. To thicken, mash the beans against the side of the pan with the back of a spoon or place in a blender and process until smooth. Blend in the cilantro.

To serve, slit each potato down the center and fluff up the pulp. With the back of a spoon, mash the potatoes down. Spoon the beans over the top.

YIELD: 4 SERVINGS

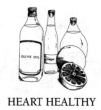

Sweet Pepper Polenta

Polenta is a dense Italian cornmeal "cake" leavened with Parmesan cheese.

$^1/_2$ teaspoon salt
$^1/_4$ teaspoon black pepper
1 cup yellow cornmeal
$^1/_4$ cup chopped sweet bell peppers (from a jar)
$^1/_4$ cup grated Parmesan or Romano cheese
1 can (15 ounces) of your favorite tomato sauce, heated

Combine $2^1/_2$ cups water, the salt, and black pepper in a sturdy saucepan and bring to a boil. Gradually stir in the cornmeal and cook for 12 to 15 minutes over low heat, stirring frequently, until thick. Remove from the heat and fold in the sweet peppers and cheese. Spread the polenta in a lightly sprayed 9-inch round pan. Allow it to reach room temperature.

Cut the polenta into wedges and place on serving plates. Spoon the tomato sauce over the top.

YIELD: 6 TO 8 SERVINGS

Pillar 7

ON THE TRAIL OF PHYTOCHEMICALS:
Vitamins of the Future

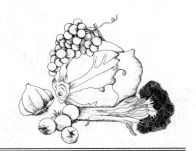

Our PARENTS AND SCHOOLTEACHERS WERE RIGHT ALL along. Vegetables and fruits really are good for us. However, few people realized just *how* good they would turn out to be. An apple a day may keep the doctor away, but to keep *chronic disease* at bay we should reach for a peach, banana, handful of berries, plenty of broccoli, tomatoes, leafy greens, and whatever else is in season. Nature has provided a pharmacy of whole foods with both curative and protective powers.

For years nutritionists have asserted that a diet rich in vegetables, fruits, grains, and legumes can reduce the risk of cancer, heart disease, and other chronic ailments. Scientists are now zeroing in on specific compounds present in plant foods that may lead the fight against chronic degenerative diseases. The trail for the holy grail has led to *phytochemicals*, the latest buzzword in health and disease prevention. An ounce of phytochemicals may be worth a pound of cure.

Phytochemicals are naturally occurring substances found abundantly in plant foods. ("Phyto" comes from the Greek word for plant, *phyton*.) Technically speaking, unlike vitamins and minerals, phytochemicals are not considered to be nutrients in the traditional sense. There is no RDA for phytochemicals (yet). However, scores of recent studies are shedding light on how phytochemicals may prevent, subdue, and even obliterate cancerous cells at several different stages of development. Without a doubt the discovery of phytochemicals is an important milestone in the ongoing quest for good health and long life.

A MULTITUDE OF PHYTOCHEMICALS OFFER PROTECTION AGAINST DISEASE

There are not one or two miracle compounds or magic bullets to this story, but a cast of hundreds, perhaps even thousands of phytochemicals that may prevent illness while promoting optimum health.

There are not one or two miracle compounds or magic bullets to this story, but a cast of hundreds, perhaps even thousands of phytochemicals that may prevent illness while promoting optimum health. Phytochemicals exist naturally in almost all vegetables, fruits, grains, and legumes. Nicknamed phytonutrients, or "phytomins" (rhymes with *vitamins*), many phytochemicals have tongue-tripping monikers like indoles, capsaicin, isoflavones, brassinin, genistein, and sulfides. While not quite household names, phytochemicals are making researchers, nutritionists, and the national media sit up and take notice.

What exactly are these plant substances that sound like they came straight out of a chemistry textbook? Phytochemicals are natural chemicals in plants that perform a variety of tasks. Certain phytochemicals help plants protect themselves against environmental dangers such as the glare of a hot sun, the withering wind, air pollution, or dehydration. Other phytochemicals help plants defend against insects, bugs, bacterial diseases, viruses, and fungi. There are phytochemicals that give plants their bright colors (like the lycopene pigment found in red tomatoes). One phytochemical, capsaicin, puts the peppery heat in hot chili peppers.

It turns out that phytochemicals may help protect *humans* from disease and toxins as well as plants. In an effort to determine exactly how phytochemicals guard against human disease, there are scores of animal studies and experiments under way all over the world. The reports coming in from laboratories sound promising and enlightening. Scientific studies have identified numerous phytochemicals that display an ability to confront, ambush, or interfere with the development of cancerous cells at every step along the way.

Reaping the Benefits of Phytochemicals

A well-balanced, plant-based diet is full of disease-fighting phytochemicals. The more phytochemicals in your diet, the merrier your health will be. Some phytochemicals increase the activity of protective enzymes and help to block cancer cells from developing. There are plant compounds that might prevent existing tumors from spreading and multiplying. Still other substances show promise by repairing damaged cells and maybe even reversing the carcinogenic process by producing "smart-bomb" enzymes that seek and destroy cancer cells.

These exciting observations are only the tip of the asparagus, so to speak, and are by no means the definitive last word. The roster of beneficial phytochemicals will continue to grow as more research comes to light. Keep in mind that any health benefits derived from phytochemicals are in the context of a well-balanced, plant-based diet high in fiber, complex carbohydrates, antioxidants, and micronutrients. Adding a sprig or two of broccoli to a meal of cheeseburgers and french fries will not significantly alter the status of your health. On the other hand, eschewing the burger and fries for a tossed green salad heaped high with vegetables and served with whole grain bread, or opting for a hearty pilaf or vegetable chili, *will* contribute to your good health and provide a mother lode of phytochemicals and other beneficial substances.

Phytochemicals on the Front Lines

Here is an overview of some breakthroughs that have garnered headlines in recent years.

Capsaicin, the plant alkaloid that gives chili peppers their spicy heat, has been credited with inhibiting the development of dangerous nitrosamines from forming during the digestive process. Capsaicin also seems to trigger the brain to release endorphins, a natural chemical that reduces pain and creates a feeling of pleasure. (This may explain the roller coaster effect felt by connoisseurs of hot-and-spicy fare—the hotter the food, the greater the allure and chili pepper "high.")

Chlorogenic Acid and *P-Coumaric,* two plant chemicals found in tomatoes, may prevent the formation of cancer cells by sabotaging the production of dangerous nitrosamines formed during the digestion process. Tomatoes are thought to contain a whopping *10,000* phytochemicals. Please pass the salsa.

Chlorophyll, the ubiquitous green pigment in plants, may offer a line of defense against cancerous cells. Chlorophyll is especially abundant in dark green vegetables (spinach, broccoli, green beans, chard, and snow peas). Chlorophyll often travels with another antioxidant pigment, beta-carotene. Greens are also excellent sources of carotenoids.

Ellagic Acid, a compound found in strawberries, grapes, apples, and raspberries, seems to fight cancer on the front line by interfering with tumor growth and blocking the production of enzymes that feed into cancer cells.

Flavonoids are found in virtually all plant foods, including berries, apples, citrus fruits, carrots, cranberries, grapes, green vegetables,

The term "phytochemicals" may sound scientific or esoteric, but the food sources are quite familiar and widely available. Cabbage, broccoli, onions, tomatoes, kale, and soy foods are phytochemical powerhouses. To fully realize the glowing health benefits of phytochemicals it is important to include these staples in your everyday meals.

and red wine. These phytochemicals may obstruct cancer-promoting hormones from attaching to normal cells and may inhibit cancer cells from spreading. This is another compelling reason to eat a variety of fruits and vegetables, not just an apple a day. Fill your plate with an orange, a carrot, leafy greens, and a handful of grapes and berries.

Indoles found in cruciferous vegetables (cabbage, broccoli, kale, collards, and cauliflower) may deter breast and prostate cancer by disarming harmful estrogen and other hormones. More good reasons to load up on crunchy cruciferous veggies.

Lutein and *Zeaxanthin,* two carotenoids found in dark leafy greens and corn, have been shown to reduce the occurrence of age-related macular degeneration (AMD), a debilitating eye condition that afflicts almost two million older adults every year. Lutein and other carotenoids are believed to protect the retina from harmful free radicals, guard against damage to the eye's macula, and ultimately delay or prevent the onset of blindness. Spinach, collards, and kale are good sources. One study found that people who ate dark leafy greens at least five times a week had *half* the risk of developing AMD compared to people who infrequently ate leafy greens.

Lycopene, the red pigment in tomatoes, has been shown to reduce the risk of prostate and stomach cancer. Lycopene is unaffected by heat and is concentrated in an assortment of canned tomato products (puréed, stewed, juiced). The red pigment is also considered to be a powerful antioxidant. (For more on lycopene, turn to Pillar 1: Unleash the Power of Antioxidants.)

Phytoestrogens (such as *genistein*) found in soy milk, tofu, and other soy foods may block the growth of new blood vessels (capillaries) leading to tumors and thwart cancer at an early stage of development. Phytoestrogens ("plant estrogens") may also protect against hormone-related cancers of the breast and prostate.

Quercetin, a potent compound found in red and yellow onions, shallots, and broccoli, may help block cancerous cells from developing. Onions are one of the most versatile staples (but avoid fried onion rings).

Resveratrol, found in the skin of grapes, may inhibit the initiation and/or growth of tumors and possibly return precancerous cells to a normal state. Resveratrol has also been linked to lowering bad cholesterol. The phytochemical is present in grapes, wine, and peanuts. Although no one has advocated dramatically increasing consumption of red wine (yet), the knowledge adds one more piece to the puzzle.

Saponin and *Isoflavones,* two more phytochemicals found in soy foods, have been linked to lowering bad cholesterol and raising the good cholesterol, thereby helping to prevent coronary heart disease. On another front, the phytochemicals may prevent cancer cells from multiplying by blocking the development of hormone-related cancers.

Sulforaphane, a compound found in broccoli, cauliflower, and kale, has been shown to increase the production of anticancer enzymes and protect against breast cancer in animal studies. Cooking might enhance the bioavailability of sulforaphane. Another good reason to eat your broccoli.

Nutrition experts are quick to point out that there is no long-term data linking specific phytochemicals to disease prevention in humans. Like many health pronouncements, the healing potential of phytochemicals is based on animal studies and lab reports. Still, health trends from around the world strongly support the health-enhancing effects of phytochemicals in the context of a plant-based diet. Study after study has shown that high consumption of phytochemical-rich foods—a wide assortment of fruits and vegetables—is associated with a reduced risk of heart disease and almost every type of cancer.

For example, Asian women have lower rates of breast cancer than Western women. The Asian diet is rich in soy foods such as tofu and soy milk. This population data supports the correlation researchers have made between consumption of phytochemical-rich soy foods and the reduced risk of certain cancers. Another study revealed that Italian men who consume tomato-based dishes at least five times a week exhibited a lower rate of prostate cancer. This conclusion reinforced the notion that something in tomatoes, most likely lycopene with other plant substances, can reduce the risk of cancer.

PHYTOCHEMICAL NUTRIENTS OFFER A SYNERGY OF PROTECTION

The emergence of phytochemicals has reinforced the need to eat a plant-based diet centered on a variety of vegetables and fruits. In the years to come we will learn more about how plant foods prevent and attack chronic disease and promote good health. There is much more to understand about how phytochemicals work together as a team with antioxidants and micronutrients present in whole foods—and perhaps with hundreds of other naturally occurring plant compounds. Clearly, there is a strong synergy between phytochemicals and other plant substances.

By the way, brace yourself for the onslaught of "phytomin pills" already hitting the stores and airwaves. There is little doubt that synthetic phytochemicals will be aggressively marketed as supplements or phytomin-enhanced pills. However, when phytochemicals are isolated as supplements they have not firmly demonstrated the same preventative powers attributed to whole foods containing the real thing. It has been said time and time again: supplements do not always mimic the health benefits linked to nutrients found in whole foods.

For instance, lutein found in spinach and flavonoids in citrus fruits may help prevent disease when derived from whole foods, but when these substances are isolated and served in a pill, all bets are off. Another example is beta-carotene, an antioxidant that is one of five hundred carotenoids present in plants such as squash and leafy greens. Beta-carotene most likely offers protection in a synergistic fashion with other carotenoids and antioxidants. Beta-carotene *in supplement form* has not lived up to its health-enhancing reputation.

It may be wishful thinking to think that one day a magic pill will be discovered and provide all of our nutrient requirements. Just pop an all-purpose super vitamin pill with a swig of water and pass the ice cream and cake. (The Food and Drug Administration recently reported that over half of all Americans take some type of vitamin supplements, and disease prevention is listed as the number-one reason.) Unfortunately, there are no easy panaceas on the horizon. In any event, a hearty and wholesome meal full of flavor and aroma can provide infinitely more pleasure than simply swallowing a vitamin pill. If anything, supplements may be a false security blanket.

Phytochemical research represents the next frontier in the study of nutrition, disease prevention, and optimum health. The discovery of vitamins ushered in the twentieth century, and it appears that phytochemicals will be the vitamins of the twenty-first century. Some day, individuals who are genetically prone to certain diseases may successfully avoid their fate by shifting their diets to phytochemical-rich foods. Just as members of a family with a history of heart disease are cautioned to avoid foods high in saturated fat, nutritional research may help women reduce their risk of breast cancer by recommending a switch from high-fat, meat-laden foods to a diet anchored with phytochemical-friendly foods such as broccoli, kale, beans, tofu, and soy milk. Families with a history of blindness will be urged to include lutein-rich leafy greens in their everyday meals. Individuals at risk for colon cancer will be encouraged early in life to eat a high-fiber diet rich with legumes, fruits, and whole grains. The possibilities for better health seem boundless.

In the future, phytochemical-rich foods may be hailed as nature's potent weapons against a range of chronic diseases.

Despite the flood of revelations and scientific breakthroughs in recent years, most Americans do not eat nearly enough phytochemical-rich foods. According to one survey, *less than 10 percent* of Americans pay heed to the well-publicized advice to eat at least five or more servings of fruits and vegetables a day. *Almost half* of all Americans do not eat *any* fruits or drink juice on a daily basis; over 20 percent rarely eat any vegetables at all. Lack of time, a surplus of unhealthy temptations, or just plain apathy can thwart the best of intentions.

In attempting to understand the mysteries of health and disease, researchers have unlocked a wellspring of secrets and solved some of the most vexing puzzles. Society is finally beginning to grasp the complex web of relationships between diet, good health, and illness. Nevertheless, if the advice goes unheeded or ignored by the masses, society has gained little.

On another note, the more things change, the more things stay the same. The basic tenets of healthy eating have not drastically changed; in fact, the refrain remains the same. To achieve optimal health and well-being, the best advice is to eat a variety of wholesome foods. Fill your plate with vegetables, grains, legumes, and fruits and avoid (or restrict) consumption of fatty animal foods and high-calorie processed foods. Let the team of phytochemicals, antioxidants, fiber, and other protective nutrients provide nourishment for both body and soul.

One of the great ironies is that our grandparents and parents extolled the virtues of fruits and vegetables during a time when grocery stores were modest pantries of canned goods and processed foods; most offered only a limited choice of fresh produce, and natural food cooperatives were dusty, scarce, and on the fringe of culture.

Fast-forward to the present: many supermarkets and natural food stores are inviting temples filled with a cornucopia of seasonal vegetables, glistening fruits, cascading leafy greens, plentiful tubers, exotic grains and legumes, and garden herbs almost all year long. From wild mushrooms to wild rice, jalapeños to mangoes, and bok choy to cilantro . . . never before in our history has there been such a copious year-round bounty of fresh produce to choose from! Phytochemical-rich foods are everywhere!

It is easy and rewarding to make the switch to a plant-based diet rich in fruits and vegetables, grains and legumes. The road to a healthy and pleasurable life runs through the produce aisle, not the pharmacy department.

It is easy and rewarding to make the switch to a plant-based diet rich in fruits and vegetables, grains and legumes. The road to a healthy and pleasurable life runs through the produce aisle, not the pharmacy department.

TWENTY WAYS TO FILL YOUR PLATE WITH FANTASTIC PHYTOCHEMICALS

1. Choose coleslaw over potato chips.
2. Add steamed broccoli to tossed salads, pasta salads, and chunky sauces.
3. Give tofu a try. Slice extra-firm tofu into strips and add to stir-fries, tomato sauce, Asian vegetable soups, pilafs, and sautéed vegetable dishes.
4. Serve your morning cereal with soy milk instead of cow's milk. If you are timid, acclimate your palate by pouring a little of both milks over the cereal. You'll gradually reduce the amount of milk you use.
5. Add cabbage to green salads, tomato soups, stir-fries, and vegetable juices.
6. Acquire a taste for hot and spicy food. Cook with fresh hot chili peppers (not canned varieties, which are more acidic) and liven up your food with fiery flavors.
7. Make a soy fruit shake in a blender with soy milk and mixed fresh fruit such as bananas, strawberries, blueberries, mangoes, kiwi fruit, and papayas.
8. Serve tomato salsa instead of sour cream, French onion dip, or tartar sauce.
9. Add kale, spinach, or collard greens to soups, chowders, pilafs, or tomato sauces.

10. Serve braised leafy greens (with lemon or wine) instead of canned vegetables.

11. Drink fresh vegetable juice four to seven days a week. If you don't own a juice extractor, go out and buy one. Fresh juice will make you feel reinvigorated, recharged, and reborn. Include a variety of vegetables and fruits such as carrots, cabbage, kale, limes, lemons, apples, parsley, beets, kiwi fruit, and celery.

12. Expand your taste for dark leafy greens. Experiment with red chard, kale, dandelion greens, turnip greens, broccoli rabe, collards, red Russian kale, bok choy, and amaranth greens.

13. Eat more fruit for dessert. Choose fruit toppings instead of chocolate frosting or whipped cream, and fresh strawberries or blueberries instead of hot fudge.

14. When dining out at Italian restaurants, order the red tomato sauce—not the cream sauce or cheesy Alfredo. Order marinara (a meatless sauce) and skip the meatballs.

15. Say good-bye to plain old white rice. Make a nourishing pilaf with sautéed onions, celery, mushrooms, garlic, sweet peppers, and whole grains.

16. Serve mashed potatoes with soy milk instead of whole milk.

17. Add blueberries, apples, or strawberries to pancakes or waffle batter. Instead of serving a fake maple syrup or butter, offer all-fruit jam, applesauce, or berries.

18. Add fresh spinach to tossed salads, potato soups, rice pots, or stir-fried dishes. Make a vow never to buy iceberg lettuce.

19. If you are a meat eater, make plans to eat at least one vegetarian dinner within the next week, even if it means going out to a vegetarian restaurant.

20. Develop a passion for garlic. Not garlic powder, garlic salt, or mashed garlic in a jar—all sorry imitations. Fresh garlic.

Add chopped garlic cloves to everything from salad dressings and dips to pasta salads and red sauces, vegetable soups, pilafs, rice dishes, bean stews, grain dishes, stir-fries, braised greens, and skillet-cooked vegetables.

PHYTOCHEMICALS IN THE KITCHEN

The names of phytochemicals may be tongue-twisters, but the many plant foods containing the compounds are as familiar as apples and oranges. (See Table 7.1.)

A Cook's Guide to Phytochemical-Rich Foods

Pages 292–295 present a guide to vegetables and fruits brimming with "phytomins."

TABLE 7.1
A Glossary to Phytochemicals

Phytochemical	Food Source	Cooking Tips
Allylic Sulfides	Onions, garlic, leeks, scallions, and chives.	Combine in aromatic base for pilafs, soups, sauces, and stews.
Anthocyanins	Cranberries, blueberries, red cabbage, beets, grapes, and pomegranates.	Include berries and cranberries in sweet breads, pancakes, muffins, and fresh juices.
Capsaicin	Hot chili peppers; the hotter the pepper, the more capsaicin present.	Remove the chili pepper seeds to temper the heat.
Coumarins	Citrus fruits, tomatoes, and parsnips.	Add lemon and limes to juice.
Ellagic acid	Strawberries, grapes, apples, and raspberries.	Toss berries with lime and serve as dessert salad.

continued

Phytochemical	Food Source	Cooking Tips
Flavonoids	Citrus fruits, tomatoes, berries, peppers, grapes, carrots, cucumbers, yams, red wine, and tea.	Eat a variety of fruits and veggies to tap into this phytochemical.
Genistein, Saponins, and Isoflavones (Phytoestrogens)	Soybeans, tofu, soy milk, and other soy foods.	Add diced tofu to sauces and stir-fries; try a soy milkshake.
Indoles	Broccoli, cabbages, kale, and cauliflower.	Quick cooking enhances bioavailability of some nutrients.
Lignans	Flaxseed, barley, wheat, and other whole grains.	Mix grains in pilafs, soups, and salads.
Lutein and Zeaxanthin	Dark leafy greens (spinach, kale, collards, chard, and mustard greens).	Braise a variety of greens with garlic, onions, and lemon. Add to soups and pilafs.
Lycopene (also an antioxidant)	Tomatoes and canned tomato products (juiced, puréed, stewed, crushed, etc.), watermelon, red grapefruit, and guava.	Use the full variety of canned tomatoes in red sauce for pasta, Creole sauce, and salsa.
P-coumaric acid and Chlorogenic acid	Tomatoes, carrots, bell peppers, pineapple, and strawberries.	Include both tomatoes and carrots in meals for maximum benefits and nutrients.
Quercetin	Onions, red onions, shallots, and broccoli.	Add chopped onions to red sauce, pilafs, bean dishes, soups, and condiments.
Resveratrol	Grapes, red wine, and peanuts.	Include grapes in salads and homemade juices; drink red wine.
Sulforaphane and Isothiocyanates	Broccoli, turnips, kale, cauliflower, and cabbage.	Buy a sturdy soup pot for these hardy staples.
Tangerertin and Nobiletin	Tangerines.	Peel and eat.

Broccoli contains a mother lode of plant nutrients including sulforaphane, indoles, and isothiocyanates. Broccoli is also a good source of vitamin C, beta-carotene, and other antioxidants. Steaming or blanching broccoli florets before eating can enhance the flavor and crunchy texture. (To maximize nutrient retention, "blanch" broccoli florets in boiling water for *only* two to three minutes until tender, not mushy.)

The world of broccoli is filled with possibilities. Toss broccoli florets into green salads, soups, stir-fries, red sauces, pasta salads, crudités platters, and vegetable medleys. Broccoli stalks can be thinly sliced and stir-fried, chopped like celery stalks for soup, or "juiced" with other vegetables in a juice extractor.

Cabbage is a haven for scores of phytochemicals including indoles, brassinin, and sulforaphane, as well as vitamin C and fiber. Add the crunchy cruciferous vegetable to wintry soups, green salads, home-made coleslaw, bean salads, stir-fries, burritos, and stews. Red cabbage (actually closer to purple) adds a splash of color to salads and contains slightly more vitamin C than green cabbage. Try them both. Adding a wedge of cabbage to fresh vegetable juice is another way to benefit from its disease-fighting benefits.

Cauliflower, another member of the cruciferous family (along with broccoli and cabbage), contains plenty of sulforaphane. Although cauliflower does not have a long culinary résumé, it can be added to soups, stews, antipasto, and marinated vegetable dishes. Add cauliflower florets to minestrone, pasta salad, sautéed mixed vegetables, and crudités platters, or toss with steamed broccoli for a side dish.

Chili Peppers contain capsaicin, a phytochemical that has no taste, odor, or flavor but puts the heat into hot peppers. The hotter the chili, the greater the level of capsaicin. Red chilies are also high in beta-carotene and vitamin C. A cornucopia of chilies add piquant flavors to almost any meal, from salsa, hummus, and pasta salads to black bean soup, hearty chili, grain or rice pilafs, spicy red sauces, and stir-fries. Look for chilies that have a smooth, taut skin and are free of blemishes or wrinkles. (For a complete glossary of chilies, turn to Pillar 5: Fire and Spice: High-Flavor, Low-Sodium Cooking with Herbs, Spices, and Chili Peppers.)

Chives have a delicate, scallionlike herbal flavor. Like other members of the allium family, chives contain allylic sulfides. Fresh chives can enhance tossed salads, dressings, light soups, and light sauces. Chopped chives also make a fanciful last-minute garnish.

Garlic has been associated with reducing the risk of heart disease, stomach cancer, and untold other ailments. Garlic contains plenty of allylic sulfides and other phytonutrients. Whether chopped, minced, or roasted, the "stinking rose" is an indispensable staple in the healthy kitchen. Garlic adds depth to pesto, salsa, hummus, vegetable soups, tomato sauces, curries, legume and grain dishes, pilafs, and vegetable entrées. To peel a clove of garlic, place it on a cutting board and give it good thump with the side of a knife or the palm of your hand. The force of the impact should loosen the skin and enable it to be easily peeled off with your fingers or a paring knife.

To roast garlic, wrap the unpeeled bulb in aluminum foil and place in a preheated 350-degree F oven for 40 to 45 minutes until tender. Remove from the oven and let cool slightly before unwrapping—the skins should easily slip off.

Store whole garlic bulbs in a ceramic bowl or jar in a cool dry place. Do not refrigerate fresh garlic—it will soften, shoot up sprouts, and develop a bitter taste. Fresh garlic should keep for several weeks if properly stored. Commercially crushed garlic sold in a jar and packed in oil is a bitter imitation of the real thing. Garlic salt should also be avoided—the flavor is pale and bordering on offensive. Garlic powder can be used, but it is not a substitute for fresh garlic.

Kale is a leafy green vegetable containing sulforaphane, isothiocaynates, and the antioxidants lutein and zeaxanthin. Chopped kale can be added to soups, curries, stir-fries, rice pots, and pasta dishes. Braised kale, when spritzed with lemon, makes a quick and easy side dish.

Leeks have a mild oniony flavor and crunchy texture. The vegetable looks like a cross between an onion and a scallion. Leeks add depth to soups and stews and are the main ingredient in vichyssoise, the potato-and-leek bisque. Like onions, leeks contain allylic sulfides, a compound that helps detoxify potential carcinogenics. When preparing leeks, remove the gritty sand particles caught between the thick leaves by soaking the stalk in a bowl of water, swishing it around, and rinsing. The whole leek can be used.

Onions are the workhorse ingredients in the healthful kitchen. Onions are believed to contain over 150 phytochemicals, including detoxifying allylic sulfides and quercetin. Onions are a lowfat way to add flavors to soups, bisques, pilafs, pasta sauces, curries, and one-pot dishes.

Yellow and white cooking onions are versatile and widely available. Red onions (really closer to purple than red) are slightly sweet and add lively colors to the pot. Large globe-shaped yellow onions (also called "Spanish" onions) are ideal for dishes prepared in large quantities. Vidalia onions (grown in Georgia), Maui onions (from Hawaii), and Bermuda onions offer sweet and succulent flavors. Despite the many varieties, most onions are interchangeable. Store onions as you store potatoes—in a cool, dark place and away from direct heat or sunshine.

Soy Foods include tofu, soy sauce, miso, tempeh, soy milk, and other processed products. Soy foods contain an abundance of phytochemicals, including cholesterol-lowering isoflavones and cancer-fighting genistein, saponin, and phytoestrogens. In addition, plant proteins found in soy foods have been linked with reduced levels of cholesterol and with reduced risk of certain cancers. (Soy milk and tofu appear separately in the glossary.)

Soy Milk, a creamy tan beverage with a nutty flavor, makes a cholesterol-free substitute for cow's milk. Soy milk can be poured over breakfast cereals and used in pancake batter, rice pudding, "creamy" sauces, baking recipes, and fruit shakes.

Tofu has a bland disposition but readily takes on any assertive flavors in a dish. Tofu blends easily into stir-fries, red sauces, puréed sauces, dips, and soups. Tofu is sold as either extra firm, firm, soft, or silken (the most soft). If you prefer a chewy texture, place extra-firm tofu in a preheated oven set at 350 degrees F and roast for about 15 minutes. Roasted tofu can be barbecued, tossed into salads or sautéed dishes, or marinated.

Tomatoes are warehouses of antioxidants, phytochemicals, and vitamin C. Fresh tomatoes and tomato-based products (canned tomatoes, stewed tomatoes, tomato paste, etc.) contain *lycopene,* the antioxidant that gives the tomato its red color. Lycopene has been linked to lower occurrences of prostate cancer. Tomatoes also contain *p-coumaric acid* and *chlorogenic acid,* two phytochemicals that may diffuse and flush out potential cancer-causing compounds such as nitrosamines.

Fresh tomatoes are important in numerous chilled dishes including tossed leafy greens, pasta and grain salads, tabbouleh, and salsa and as a garnish for sandwiches. Canned tomato products form the basis of myriad pasta sauces, pizza, vegetable soups, bean soups, Creole sauce, ratatouille, and other healthy dishes.

Turnips are bulbous roots with a purple band around the top. Turnips have a crisp white flesh and mild radish-mustardy flavor. As a member of the cruciferous family, turnips contain isothiocyanates. Add turnips to hearty soups and stews along with potatoes and other root vegetables. Turnip greens can also be used; they are rich in antioxidants (although they have a bitter mustard flavor).

Watercress has green oval leaves with a peppery herbal flavor. Watercress contains isothiocyanates. The tender green adds zest to leafy salads, dressings, tabbouleh, soups, pasta dishes, potato salads, and chowders.

SIGNATURE RECIPES FOR THE PHYTOCHEMICAL-RICH, HEALTHY DIET

Spicy Cabbage Sofrito

Cranberry Bog Chutney

Cabbage Patch Bisque

Hot Cabbage Gumbo

Sweet Corn and Broccoli Chowder

Mizuna Salad with Caramelized Onions and Sweet Peppers

Lemony Coleslaw

Wheat Garden Salad with Watercress

Pasta Marinara with Broccoli

Green Rice Pilaf with Watercress

Eggplant and Tomato Ragout with Tofu

Wild Mushroom Stir-Fry with Tofu

Green Spinach Soup

Leafy Turnip Tureen

Mashed Root Vegetables

Onion Pumpkin Bread with Sunflower Seeds

Tofu Kiwi-Berry Smoothie

Additional health benefits are noted with each recipe.

Spicy Cabbage Sofrito

This is a chunky sauce of cabbage, peppers, and tomatoes. Serve it as a topping for pilaf, pasta, or rice dishes.

1   tablespoon canola oil
1   medium yellow onion, diced
1   green pepper, seeded and diced
2   cups coarsely chopped cabbage
2   large cloves garlic, minced
1   jalapeño pepper, seeded and minced
1   can (14 ounces) stewed tomatoes
1   can (14 ounces) tomato purée
2   teaspoons dried oregano
$^1/_2$ teaspoon black pepper

In a medium saucepan heat the oil over medium-high heat. Add the onion, bell pepper, cabbage, garlic, and jalapeño pepper and cook, stirring, for about 6 minutes. Add the stewed tomatoes, tomato purée, oregano, and pepper and cook over medium-low heat until the cabbage is tender, about 15 to 20 minutes, stirring occasionally.

Spoon the sofrito over rice or pasta dishes.

YIELD: 6 SERVINGS

Cranberry Bog Chutney

FIBER

HEART HEALTHY

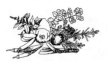

FIRE AND SPICE

This sweet-and-tart condiment is a glistening blend of autumn fruit, apple cider, vinegar, and aromatic spices.

12 ounces fresh or frozen cranberries
2 red apples, diced (do not peel)
1 large yellow onion, diced
4 cloves garlic, minced
1 tablespoon minced ginger root
$3/4$ cup brown sugar
$1/2$ cup raisins or 1 cup chopped dried apricots
$1^{1}/2$ cups red wine vinegar
1 cup apple cider
$1/2$ teaspoon black pepper
$1/2$ teaspoon cumin
$1/2$ teaspoon salt
$1/4$ teaspoon ground cloves

Combine all of the ingredients in a large, nonreactive saucepan. Cook over medium-low heat, stirring occasionally, for 25 to 30 minutes until the mixture has a jamlike consistency. Allow the chutney to cool to room temperature.

Serve the chutney warm or refrigerate for later. If kept refrigerated, the chutney should keep for several weeks. Serve as a companion to rice dishes, curries, scones, or grain pilafs.

YIELD: 6 TO 8 SERVINGS

HELPFUL HINT

Serve the chutney with barbecued vegetables or chicken.

Cabbage Patch Bisque

This soup is brimming with good-for-you phytochemicals, antioxidants, and fine flavors. A touch of vinegar coaxes out the mild flavors of cabbage and potatoes.

ANTIOXIDANTS

1   tablespoon canola oil
1   medium yellow onion, diced
1   large stalk celery, diced
3   or 4 cloves garlic, minced
4   cups vegetable broth or water
2   cups diced white potatoes
2   cups coarsely chopped cabbage
1/2   teaspoon salt
1/2   teaspoon white pepper
2   cups coarsely chopped kale
1   can (15 ounces) white kidney beans, drained
1   cup soy milk or skim milk
1/4   cup chopped fresh parsley
1   to 2 tablespoons wine vinegar

FIBER

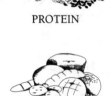

PROTEIN

In a large saucepan heat the oil over medium heat. Add the onion, celery, and garlic and cook, stirring, for about 4 minutes. Add the broth, potatoes, cabbage, salt, and pepper and bring to a simmer. Cook for 10 minutes over medium heat, stirring occasionally. Stir in the kale and beans and cook for 10 to 15 minutes more until the potatoes are tender. Stir in the soy milk and parsley.

POWER EATING

Transfer the soup (in batches) to a food processor fitted with a steel blade or to a blender and process for 5 to 10 seconds until smooth. Swirl in the vinegar.

Ladle the bisque into bowls and serve with warm crusty bread.

YIELD: 6 SERVINGS

Hot Cabbage Gumbo

This zesty meatless gumbo is abundant with spicy flavors and hearty textures. Cabbage, tomatoes, and brown rice provide an assortment of nutrients.

ANTIOXIDANTS

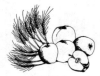

FIBER

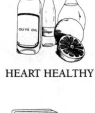

HEART HEALTHY

PROTEIN

1   tablespoon canola oil
1   medium yellow onion, diced
1   green or red bell pepper, seeded and diced
1   large stalk celery, chopped
3 or 4 cloves garlic, minced
5   cups vegetable stock or water
1   can (14 ounces) stewed tomatoes
2   cups coarsely chopped cabbage
1   can (15 ounces) small red beans, drained
$^1/_2$ cup brown rice
$^1/_4$ cup tomato purée or paste
1   tablespoon dried oregano
1   teaspoon dried thyme
$^1/_2$ teaspoon black pepper
$^1/_2$ teaspoon salt
$^1/_4$ teaspoon cayenne pepper

In a large saucepan heat the oil over medium heat. Add the onion, bell pepper, celery, and garlic and cook, stirring, for 5 to 7 minutes. Stir in the vegetable stock or water, stewed tomatoes, cabbage, beans, rice, tomato purée or paste, oregano, thyme, pepper, salt, and cayenne and bring to a simmer. Cook over medium heat for 35 minutes until the rice is tender, stirring occasionally.

Remove from the heat and let stand for 5 minutes. Ladle the gumbo into soup bowls and serve with warm wheat bread or corn-bread.

YIELD: 6 SERVINGS

HELPFUL HINT

Chicken or fish stock can be used in place of the vegetable stock.

HEART HEALTHY

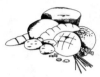

POWER EATING

Sweet Corn and Broccoli Chowder

This healthful version of corn chowder is especially appetizing when made with corn kernels cut fresh off the cob.

1 tablespoon canola oil
1 medium yellow onion, chopped
1 red bell pepper, seeded and diced
2 or 3 cloves garlic, minced
4 cups vegetable broth
2 cups diced white potatoes
1 teaspoon dried thyme
1 teaspoon salt
$^1/_2$ teaspoon black pepper
12 broccoli florets (about 1 small head)
2 cups corn kernels
$^1/_4$ cup chopped fresh parsley
1 cup lowfat milk

In a large saucepan heat the oil over medium-high heat. Add the onion, bell pepper, and garlic and cook, stirring, for 5 minutes. Add the broth, potatoes, thyme, salt, and pepper and bring to a simmer. Cook for 12 to 15 minutes over medium heat, stirring occasionally.

Stir in the broccoli, corn, and parsley and cook for 8 minutes more. Stir in the milk and return to a gentle simmer. Let the chowder stand for 5 to 10 minutes before serving. To thicken, either mash the potatoes against the side of the pan with a large spoon or purée in a blender about 2 cups of soup and return to the pan. Ladle the chowder into bowls and serve with warm bread.

YIELD: 6 SERVINGS

Mizuna Salad with Caramelized Onions and Sweet Peppers

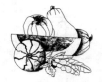

ANTIOXIDANTS

The sweet essence of caramelized onions brings out the mustardlike nuance of Japanese mizuna greens.

1 tablespoon canola oil
2 medium yellow onions, sliced into thin slivers
1 large red bell pepper, seeded and cut into thin strips
1 tablespoon balsamic vinegar
1 tablespoon brown sugar
1 bunch mizuna greens, rinsed and coarsely chopped
2 ounces alfalfa sprouts
1 tomato, cut into wedges

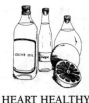

HEART HEALTHY

In a large skillet heat the oil over medium-high heat. Add the slivered onions and pepper and cook, stirring, for 7 minutes until lightly browned. Reduce the heat to low and stir in the vinegar and sugar. Cook, stirring, for 2 minutes more.

Meanwhile, arrange the mizuna, sprouts, and tomato on salad plates. Using tongs, place the onion mixture over the top. Serve the greens as a first course or side dish.

YIELD: 4 SERVINGS

HELPFUL HINT

Mizuna is available at well-stocked supermarkets and Asian grocery stores.

Lemony Coleslaw

ANTIOXIDANTS

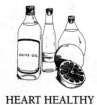

HEART HEALTHY

This inviting alternative to traditional mayonnaise-based coleslaw has a tangy personality.

2 cups shredded red cabbage
2 carrots, shredded
1 small red onion, chopped
1 small cucumber, chopped (peeled if waxed)
2 to 3 tablespoons chopped fresh parsley
Juice of 1 large lemon
1 tablespoon canola oil
$1/2$ teaspoon celery seeds
$1/2$ teaspoon black pepper
$1/2$ teaspoon salt

Combine all of the ingredients in a mixing bowl and refrigerate for 30 minutes or overnight. Serve the coleslaw as a light side dish or salad.

YIELD: 4 SERVINGS

Wheat Garden Salad
with Watercress

Watercress adds a nice herbal zing to this tabbouleh-style salad. It makes a tangy salad or light filling for pita bread.

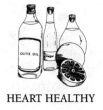

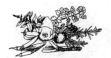

1 cup bulgur
1$\frac{1}{2}$ cups boiling water
2 large scallions, chopped
$\frac{1}{2}$ cup chopped fresh parsley
$\frac{1}{2}$ cup watercress leaves
4 plum tomatoes, diced
1 cucumber, chopped (peeled if waxed)
Juice of 2 lemons
3 to 4 tablespoons olive oil
2 cloves garlic, minced (optional)
$\frac{1}{2}$ teaspoon black pepper
$\frac{1}{2}$ teaspoon salt

Combine the bulgur and boiling water in a pan, cover, and let sit for 20 minutes until all of the water is absorbed.

In a mixing bowl, combine the bulgur with the remaining ingredients and toss thoroughly. Chill for at least 1 hour before serving.

Serve the salad over a bed of leafy greens with warm pita bread.

YIELD: 4 SERVINGS

HELPFUL HINT

For a variation, add a little crumbled feta cheese or chick-peas.

Pasta Marinara with Broccoli

This simple dish of pasta and tomato sauce is improved with the presence of broccoli, beans, and herbs.

ANTIOXIDANTS

FIBER

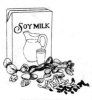

PROTEIN

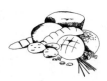

POWER EATING

1 tablespoon canola oil
1 medium yellow onion, diced
2 large cloves garlic, minced
1 can (28 ounces) plum tomatoes
2 tablespoons chopped fresh parsley
2 teaspoons dried oregano
1 teaspoon dried basil
$^1\!/_2$ teaspoon black pepper
$^1\!/_2$ teaspoon salt
8 ounces bow tie pasta
1 small bunch broccoli, cut into florets
1 cup cooked red kidney beans
$^1\!/_4$ cup grated Parmesan cheese (optional)

In a large saucepan heat the oil over medium heat. Add the onion and garlic and cook, stirring, for 4 minutes until translucent. Add the plum tomatoes, parsley, oregano, basil, pepper, and salt and bring to a simmer. Cook for 15 to 20 minutes over low heat, stirring occasionally.

Meanwhile, in a large saucepan bring 3$^1\!/_2$ quarts of water to a boil over medium-high heat. Place the pasta in the boiling water, stir, and return to a boil. Cook for 8 minutes and then stir in the broccoli florets. Cook for 3 to 5 minutes more, stirring occasionally, until the pasta is al dente. Drain the pasta and broccoli in a colander. Transfer to a large warm serving dish.

Transfer the red sauce to a food processor fitted with a steel blade or to a blender and process for about 5 seconds until smooth. Return the sauce to the pan and stir in the beans. Return to a gentle simmer over medium heat.

Ladle the sauce over the pasta and broccoli. If desired, sprinkle the Parmesan cheese over the top.

YIELD: 4 SERVINGS

Green Rice Pilaf with Watercress

ANTIOXIDANTS

HEART HEALTHY

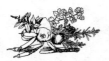

FIRE AND SPICE

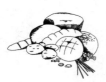

POWER EATING

Here's a way to combine plenty of phytochemical-rich greens and herbs with sturdy grains and vegetables.

1   tablespoon canola oil
1   medium yellow onion, diced
1   green bell pepper, seeded and diced
3   or 4 cloves garlic, minced
1   large jalapeño pepper, seeded and minced (optional)
2½ cups chopped fresh spinach or kale
2   cups diced sweet potatoes or butternut squash (peeled)
1½ cups long grain white or brown rice
1½ teaspoons ground cumin
½   teaspoon salt
½   teaspoon black pepper
½   cup watercress leaves, rinsed
4   whole scallions, chopped

In a medium saucepan heat the oil over medium heat. Add the onion, bell pepper, garlic, and jalapeño and cook, stirring, for 6 minutes. Stir in the spinach or kale and cook, stirring, until the greens are wilted, about 3 minutes. Stir in 3¼ cups water, the sweet potatoes or squash, rice, cumin, salt, and pepper and bring to a simmer. Cover and cook over medium-low heat until the rice and squash are tender, about 20 minutes (if using brown rice, about 30 minutes). Fluff the rice and stir in the watercress and scallions. Let stand (still covered) for about 5 minutes before serving.

YIELD: 6 SERVINGS

HELPFUL HINT

This makes a nourishing side dish to burritos, chicken, or grilled seafood.

Eggplant and Tomato Ragout with Tofu

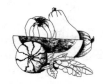

ANTIOXIDANTS

For a nourishing meal, serve this chunky vegetable stew over rice, pasta, or quinoa.

1 tablespoon canola oil
1 medium yellow onion, diced
1 green bell pepper, seeded and diced
2 cups diced eggplant
3 or 4 cloves garlic, minced
1 can (28 ounces) plum tomatoes
1 can (11 ounces) corn kernels, drained
$^1/_4$ pound extra-firm tofu, diced
2 teaspoons dried oregano
1 teaspoon chili powder
$^1/_2$ teaspoon black pepper
$^1/_2$ teaspoon salt

HEART HEALTHY

PROTEIN

In a large saucepan heat the oil over medium heat. Add the onion, bell pepper, eggplant, and garlic and cook, stirring, over medium heat for about 8 minutes. Stir in the plum tomatoes, corn, tofu, oregano, chili powder, pepper, and salt and bring to a simmer. Cook for 15 to 20 minutes over medium-low heat, stirring occasionally.

Let stand for 5 to 10 minutes before serving. Ladle the "ragout" into bowls and serve with rice, pasta, or grains.

YIELD: 4 SERVINGS

Wild Mushroom Stir-Fry with Tofu

ANTIOXIDANTS

HEART HEALTHY

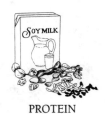

PROTEIN

Broccoli and mushrooms—especially woodsy wild mushrooms— share a natural affinity for each other. They team up with success in this quick-and-easy stir-fry.

2 teaspoons peanut oil or canola oil
8 ounces button mushrooms, sliced
4 ounces fresh oyster or shiitake mushrooms, sliced
1 red bell pepper, seeded and cut into thin strips
1 hot chili pepper, seeded and minced (optional)
2 teaspoons minced ginger root
12 broccoli florets (about 1 small head)
1/4 pound extra-firm tofu, cut into matchsticks
2 teaspoons cornstarch
1/4 cup low-sodium soy sauce
1 to 2 teaspoons toasted sesame oil
1/2 teaspoon black pepper
2 ounces bean sprouts (optional)

In a large wok or skillet heat the oil. Add the mushrooms, bell pepper, hot pepper, and ginger and stir-fry for 5 to 7 minutes over medium-high heat. Add the broccoli and tofu and stir-fry for 4 to 6 minutes more until the broccoli is tender.

Meanwhile in a small bowl combine the cornstarch and 2 teaspoons water to form a slurry.

Slide the vegetables away from the center of the wok and form a ring around a "well." Add the soy sauce, sesame oil, and black pepper to the well and bring to a simmer. To thicken, whisk in the cornstarch slurry and return to a simmer. Coat the vegetables with the thickened soy sauce.

Serve the vegetables over cooked rice or noodles. To garnish, shower the sprouts over the top.

YIELD: 2 SERVINGS AS A MAIN COURSE OR 4 AS A SIDE DISH

HELPFUL HINT

For a nutritious variation, add $1/2$ cup chopped cabbage or carrots to the wok along with the broccoli.

Green Spinach Tureen

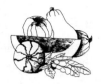

ANTIOXIDANTS

HEART HEALTHY

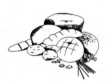

POWER EATING

Spinach and potatoes meld seamlessly together in this satisfying bisque.

1 tablespoon olive oil
1 medium yellow onion, diced
4 cloves garlic, minced
8 cups coarsely chopped fresh spinach
2 cups peeled, diced white potatoes
$^1/_2$ teaspoon dried thyme
$^1/_2$ teaspoon salt
$^1/_2$ teaspoon white pepper
$^1/_4$ teaspoon ground nutmeg
$^1/_4$ cup chopped fresh parsley

In a large saucepan heat the oil over medium heat. Add the onion and garlic and cook, stirring, for 4 minutes. Add the spinach and cook, stirring, until wilted, about 2 minutes. Add 4 cups water, the potatoes, thyme, salt, pepper, and nutmeg and bring to a simmer. Cook until the potatoes are tender, about 20 minutes, stirring occasionally. Stir in the parsley.

Transfer the soup to a blender or a food processor fitted with a steel blade and process until puréed, about 10 seconds. Ladle the soup into bowls and serve hot.

YIELD: 4 SERVINGS

Leafy Turnip Tureen

This wintry cauldron is teeming with protective nutrients and energy-supplying carbohydrates.

FIBER

- 1 tablespoon olive oil
- 1 medium yellow onion, chopped
- 2 or 3 cloves garlic, minced
- 4 cups water or vegetable broth
- 2 cups diced white potatoes
- 2 medium turnips, peeled and diced
- 1/2 teaspoon salt
- 1/2 teaspoon ground white pepper
- 2 cups chopped turnip greens
- 1 can (15 ounces) white kidney beans, drained
- 1/4 cup chopped fresh parsley

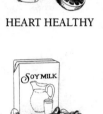

HEART HEALTHY

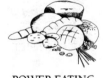

PROTEIN

In a large saucepan heat the oil over medium heat. Add the onion and garlic and cook, stirring, for about 4 minutes. Add the water, potatoes, turnips, salt, and pepper and bring to a simmer. Cook for 20 minutes over medium heat, stirring occasionally. Stir in the turnip greens, beans, and parsley and cook for 10 to 15 minutes more. Turn off the heat and let stand for about 10 minutes. To thicken, mash the potatoes against the side of the pan with the back of a spoon.

POWER EATING

Ladle the soup into bowls and serve with warm crusty bread.

YIELD: 6 SERVINGS

HELPFUL HINT

Chicken stock can be used in place of water.

Mashed Root Vegetables

This is a great way to enjoy a variety of root vegetables.

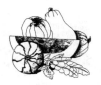

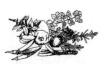

2   teaspoons canola oil
1   medium yellow onion, diced
2   large cloves garlic, minced
2   medium turnips, scrubbed and diced
2   large carrots, peeled and diced
1   medium beet, scrubbed and diced
$^1/_2$ teaspoon salt
$^1/_2$ teaspoon black pepper
$^1/_4$ cup chopped fresh parsley
$^1/_4$ cup watercress leaves

In a medium saucepan heat the oil over medium-high heat. Add the onion and garlic and cook, stirring, for 3 to 4 minutes. Add the turnips, carrots, beet, 2 cups water, salt, and pepper and bring to a simmer. Cook until the vegetables are tender, about 25 to 30 minutes, stirring occasionally.

Transfer the vegetables and liquid to a food processor fitted with a steel blade or to a blender and process until creamy, about 5 seconds. Transfer the purée to a serving bowl and top with the parsley and watercress. Serve as a side dish.

YIELD: 4 SERVINGS

Onion Pumpkin Bread
with Sunflower Seeds

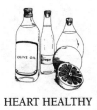

This delicious and moist sweet bread is addictive and healthful. It is easy to go overboard, and a challenge to eat just one slice.

ANTIOXIDANTS

HEART HEALTHY

1½ cups all-purpose flour
½ cup whole wheat flour
1 tablespoon baking powder
1 teaspoon salt
1 teaspoon ground ginger
½ teaspoon black pepper
½ cup canola oil
½ cup brown sugar
¼ cup molasses
1 large egg and 1 egg white
½ cup soy milk or lowfat milk
1 can (15 ounces) mashed pumpkin
1 large sweet onion, finely chopped
    (such as Maui, Vidalia, or Bermuda)
¼ cup roasted sunflower seeds (unsalted)

Preheat the oven to 375 degrees F.

In a mixing bowl, combine all of the dry ingredients. In a separate bowl whisk together the oil, brown sugar, molasses, eggs, and milk. Blend in the pumpkin and onion. Gradually fold the dry ingredients into the wet batter.

Pour the batter into two lightly greased 8-inch-by-4-inch loaf pans. Sprinkle the sunflower seeds over the top. Bake for 50 to 60 minutes, until a toothpick inserted in the center comes out clean. Let the bread cool slightly before serving.

YIELD: 2 LOAVES

Tofu Kiwi-Berry Smoothie

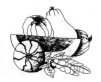

ANTIOXIDANTS

This fruity and creamy treat is made with silken tofu, an ultra-soft version of tofu. It is a healthful liquid snack good for any time of day.

HEART HEALTHY

2 cups silken tofu (soft)
2 cups strawberries or blueberries (thawed, if frozen)
2 kiwi fruits, peeled and diced
2 bananas, diced
$1/4$ teaspoon ground nutmeg

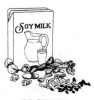

PROTEIN

Combine all of the ingredients in a blender and process for 5 to 10 seconds until creamy. Pour into cold glasses and serve as a beverage or dessert.

YIELD: 2 SERVINGS

Suggested Reference Books

Anderson, Jean, and Barbara Deskins. *The Nutrition Bible*. New York: William Morrow and Company, Inc., 1995.

Barnard, Neil. *Food For Life: How the New Four Food Groups Can Save Your Life*. New York: Harmony Books, 1993.

Brody, Jane. *Jane Brody's Good Food Book: Living the High Carbohydrate Way*. New York: Bantam Books, 1987.

Carper, Jean. *Stop Aging Now!: The Ultimate Plan for Staying Young and Reversing the Aging Process*. New York: HarperCollins, 1996.

———. *Food—Your Miracle Medicine*. New York: HarperCollins, 1993.

Gershoff, Stanley. *The Tufts University Guide to Total Nutrition*. New York: Harper & Row, 1990.

Jacobi, Dana. *The Natural Health Cookbook*. New York: Simon & Schuster, 1995.

Kleiner, Susan, and Maggie Greenwood-Robinson. *High Performance Nutrition*. New York: John Wiley & Sons, Inc., 1996.

Kronhausen, Eberhard, and Phyllis Kronhausen. *Formula For Life: The Anti-Oxidant, Free-Radical Detoxification Program*. New York: William Morrow and Company, Inc., 1989.

McDougall, John. *The McDougall Program: Twelve Days to Dynamic Health*. New York: NAL Books, The Penguin Group, 1990.

Margen, Sheldon, and Editors of the University of California, Berkeley, Wellness Letter. *The Wellness Encyclopedia of Food and Nutrition*. New York: Rebus, 1992.

Miller, Mark, and John Harrison. *The Great Chile Book*. Berkeley, California: Ten Speed Press, 1991.

Mindell, Earl. *Earl Mindell's Soy Miracle*. New York: Fireside, 1995.

Ornish, Dean. *Eat More, Weigh Less*. New York: HarperCollins, 1993.

Page, Helen Cassidy, and John Speer Schroeder. *The Stanford Life Plan for a Healthy Heart*. San Francisco: Chronicle Books, 1996.

Reader's Digest Live Longer Cookbook. Pleasantville, New York: Reader's Digest Association, Inc., 1992.

Solomon, Jay. *Lean Bean Cuisine*. Rocklin, California: Prima Publishing, 1995.

Solomon, Jay. *Vegetarian Rice Cuisine*. Rocklin, California: Prima Publishing, 1996.

Spiller, Gene A. *Eat Your Way to Better Health*. Rocklin, California: Prima Publishing, 1996.

Recipe Index

General Index

A

Acorn squash, 23
Adzuki beans, 57–58
Age-related macular degeneration
  (AMD), 8, 283
Aji dulce chilies, 204
Alcohol consumption, 5
Allspice, 198
Allylic sulfides, 290
Alpha-carotene, 8, 9
Amaranth
  grains, 155, 157–158, 248
  greens, 17
Amino acids, 150
  in legumes, 154–155
  protein and, 153–154
Anaheim chilies, 203
Anasazi beans, 58
Angioplasty, 94
Animal foods. *See also* Protein
  cholesterol and, 99
  fiber in, 48
Antacids, 150
Anthosyanins, 290
Antioxidants, 1–25
  beta-carotene, 7–8
  boosting intake of, 14–15

carotenoids, 7–8, 9
  in carrots, 15
  in dark leafy greens, 15–20
  free radicals and, 4
  lutein, 7–8
  lycopene, 10–11
  rainbow of foods, 11–13
  selenium, 11
  understanding potential of, 2–4
  vitamin C, 5–7
  vitamin E, 9–10
  from whole foods, 13–14
Appetize, 109
Arborio rice, 243, 245
Aromatics, 205–206
Arteriosclerosis, 94
Arugula, 118, 194
Ascorbic acid. *See* Vitamin C

B

Baby bok choy, 18
Balsamic vinegar, 112
Barley, 248
Barnard, Neal, 151
Basil, 194
Basmati rice, 245

Cellulose, 48
Champagne vinegar, 112
Chard, 18
Chervil, 194
Chick-peas, 58
Chicory, 118
Chili peppers, 185–187, 200–205
    allure of, 201–202
    hot sauces, 205
    phytochemicals in, 292–293
    tips for cooking with, 202–203
    types of, 202–204
Chili Powder, 201
Chinese Five Spice, 201
Chinese parsley, 195
Chipotle peppers, 203
Chives, 195
    phytochemicals in, 293
Chlorogenic acid, 282
Chlorophyll, 16, 282
Cholesterol. *See also* Low-
        cholesterol cooking
    animal protein–cholesterol
        connection, 106–107
    description of, 93–94
    dietary cholesterol, 96–97
    fiber and, 49
    free radicals and, 3
    healthy alternative recipes, 110
    heart disease and, 103–104
    high cholesterol readings, 94–95
    isoflavones, 284
    reducing cholesterol in diet,
        107–109
    resveratrol, 284
    role of, 93–94
    saponin, 284
    in soy foods, 159
    tips on controlling, 98–99
    trans fatty acids and, 104, 106
    truth about, 91–93
    vitamin E and, 9
Cider vinegar, 112

Cigarette smoking. *See* Smoking
Cilantro, 195
Cinnamon, 198
Citrus fruits, 21
Citrus juices, 114–115
Collagen, vitamin C and, 5
Collard greens, 18
Colon cancer
    animal protein and, 149
    fiber and, 50
Columbus, Christopher, 196
Complex carbohydrates, 233–253
    difference between simple carbo-
        hydrates and, 242
    food sources for, 236–237,
        239–240
    merits of, 234–235
    in pasta, 249–251
    in potatoes, 251–253
    rice, 241–246
    tips for high-energy diet,
        240–241
    weight loss and, 239
    in whole grains, 246–249
Constipation, fiber preventing, 49
Converted rice, 245–246
Coriander, 195
Corn, 248
    complete proteins with, 154
Corn oil, 113
Corn syrup, 238
Coronary artery disease. *See* Heart
        disease
Cottage cheese, lowfat, 116
Coumarins, 290
Couscous, 248–249
    whole wheat, 61–62
Cracked wheat, 61, 248
Cranberry beans, 58
Cruciferous vegetables, 283
Cumin, 198–199
Curly endive, 118
Curry Powder, 201

D

Dairy products, lowfat, 115–116
Dandelion greens, 19
Dark leafy greens
    antioxidants in, 15–20
    fiber in, 55
    iron in, 152
    low-cholesterol cooking with,
        116–119
    phytochemicals in, 289
    preparation tips, 117
    tips for preparing, 16–17
Delicata squash, 24
Dietary cholesterol, 96–97
Dietary fats, 96
    excess dietary fat, 100–102
    food sources, 100
    reducing fats in diet, 107–109
    types of, 101–103
Dietary fiber. *See* Fiber
Dill, 195
Diverticulosis, fiber and, 50
DNA, free radicals and, 3
Dried herbs, 193

E

E. coli, 151
Elimination process, 49
Ellagic acid, 282, 290
Endorphins, 202
Energy diet tips, 240–241
Escarole, 18
Exercise, blood pressure and, 192

F

Fake fat substitutes, 109–110
Family history, 5
Fats, 89–90. *See also* Cholesterol;
        Dietary fats
    differences among, 101
    healthy alternative recipes, 110

heart disease and, 103–104
lipids, 99–100
reducing fats in diet, 107–109
Fatty acids, 99
Fiber, 47–63
    in animal foods, 48
    benefits of, 48, 52–53
    crisis in eating, 53–54
    facts on, 49
    food sources for, 52, 56–63
    insoluble fiber, 51
    jump-starting diet with, 56
    in legumes. *See also* Beans
    low-fiber–containing foods, 53
    soluble fiber, 51–52
    supplements and pills, 54
    tips on boosting fiber intake,
        55–56
    virtues of, 49–50
Fines herbes, 194, 197
Flavonoids, 282–283, 291
Flavored vinegars, 112
Flour, whole wheat, 63
Food-related illnesses, 151
Free radicals, 3
    antioxidants and, 4
    beta-carotene and, 8
Freezing foods and vitamin C, 6
French chicory, 19
Fresh herbs, 193
Fried foods, 105, 108
Frisee, 19, 118
Fructose, 238
Fruits
    fructose in, 239
    iron in, 152

G

Garam Masala, 201
Garbanzo beans, 58
Garlic, 205–206, 289–290
    phytochemicals in, 293

Genistein, 283, 291
  in soy foods, 159
Ginger root, 206
Glucose, 235
  complex carbohydrates and, 237
  insulin and, 235
  simple carbohydrates and, 238
Glycogen, 235
Golden Hubbard squash, 24
Grains. *See* Whole grains
Grapefruits, 21
Great Northern beans, 59
Green chard. *See* Chard
Green leaf lettuce, 118
Green peppercorns, 198–199
Ground red pepper, 198–199
Gungo peas, 59

H

Habanero chilies, 203
Heartburn, 150
Heart disease, 91–92
  arteriosclerosis, 94
  cholesterol and, 103–104
  fats and, 103–104
  fiber and, 50
  hypertension and, 188
  plaque, 94
  protein and, 149
  saturated fats and, 102, 103–104
Hemicellulose, 48
Hemorrhoids, fiber and, 49, 50
Herbes de Provence, 197
Herbs, 185–187, 192–196
  blends of, 196, 197
  tips for cooking with, 193–194
High-density lipoprotein (HDL), 95
High-energy diet tips, 240–241
Horseradish, 206
Hot sauces, 205
Hydrogenation, 104
Hypertension, 186–187, 188

I

Iceberg lettuce, 16
Idaho potatoes, 252
Immune system
  vitamin C and, 5
  vitamin E and, 9
Indigestion, 150
Indoles, 283, 291
Insoluble fiber, 51
Insulin, 235
Iron, sources of, 152
Isoflavones, 284, 291
  in soy foods, 159
Isothiocyanates, 291
Italian seasonings, 197

J

Jalapeño peppers, 203
Jasmati rice, 245
Jasmine rice, 245
Juices in low-cholesterol cooking,
    114–115

K

Kabocha squash, 24
Kale, 19
  phytochemicals in, 293
Kidney beans, 59
Kiwi fruit, 21

L

Laxatives, 54
Leafy greens. *See* Dark leafy greens
Leeks, phytochemicals in, 294
Legumes, 56–60. *See also* Beans
  amino acids in, 154–155
  cooking tips, 57
  fiber from, 52
  steps in bean routine, 60
Lemon grass, 206

P

Papain, 22
Papaya, 22
Paprika, 198–199
Parboiled rice, 245–246
Parsley, 195
Pasta
  complex carbohydrates in, 240,
    249–251
  do's and don'ts of, 252
  guide to, 250–251
  quinoa spaghetti, 251
  spelt pasta, 160
  spelt spaghetti, 251
  whole wheat pasta, 63
  whole wheat spaghetti, 251
Pat soi, 18
P-coumaric acid, 282, 291, 295
Peanut oil, 114
Pearled barley, 248
Pectin, 48
Peppercorns, 198–199
Pepperoncinis, 204
Physicians Committee for Respon-
    sible Medicine, 151
Phytochemicals, 279–295
  disease protection, 280–285
  food sources for, 290–291
  guide to cooking with,
    290–295
  overview of, 282–285
  reaping benefits of, 281–282
  in soy foods, 159
  synthetic phytochemicals,
    285–286
  tips for using, 288–290
Phytoestrogens, 283, 291
  in soy foods, 159
Phytomins, 280
Pigeon peas, 59
Pineapple, 22
Pink peppercorns, 198–199
Pinto beans, 59

Plaque, 94
  oxidation process, 98
Poblano chilies, 204
Polyunsaturated fats, 96, 102–103
Potassium, 192
Potatoes
  complex carbohydrates in, 240,
    251–253
  three-step method to baking
    potatoes, 253
  tips on preparing, 253
Processed foods, fiber in, 54
Protein
  amino acids and, 153–154
  animal protein–cholesterol
    connection, 106–107
  comparison of plant and animal
    proteins, 157
  cook's guide to plant proteins,
    157–161
  creating complete proteins, 156
  high protein intake, 152
  myths, 147–161
  plant proteins, 155–156
  problems with, 149–151
  vegetable proteins, 154–155
Pumpkin, 24

Q

Quercetin, 284, 291
Quinoa, 249
  amino acids in, 155
  protein in, 158–159
  spaghetti, 251

R

Radicchio, 119
Rapeseed oil, 113
Rapini, 18
Red chard. *See* Chard
Red Fresno chilies, 204

Southern greens, 19
Soybeans, 59, 154–155
Soy foods
  amino acids in, 155
  breast cancer and, 285
  phytochemicals in, 294
  protein in, 152, 159
  vitamin B-12 in, 153
Soy milk
  phytochemicals in, 294
  protein in, 159–160
Soy sauce, low-sodium, 191
Spaghetti. *See* Pasta
Spelt, 249
  protein in, 160
  spaghetti, 251
Spices, 185–187, 196–200
  blends, 200, 201
  roasting spices, 198
  whole and ground, 197
Spinach, 19–20, 119
Split peas, 59, 160
Squash, 22–25
Starches. *See* Complex carbo-
  hydrates
Star fruit, 22
Sugar. *See also* Simple carbo-
  hydrates
  foods containing, 238
Sugar loaf squash, 25
Sugar pie pumpkins, 24
Sulforaphane, 284, 291
Sweet dumpling squash, 25
Sweet potatoes, 20
Swiss chard. *See* Chard
Synthetic fats, 109–110
Synthetic pills, 13

T
Tabasco sauce, 205
Tangerertin, 291
Tangerines, 21, 291

Tarragon, 196
Tat soi, 18
Tempeh, protein in, 160
Thyme, 196
Tocopherol. *See* Vitamin E
Tofu
  phytochemicals in, 288, 295
  protein in, 160–161
Tomatoes, 20–21
  phytochemicals in, 282, 295
Toxins, 3–4
Trans fats, 96, 104
  avoidance of, 111
  inventory of, 107
Trans fatty acids, 104, 106
Tropical fruits, 21–22
Tryptophan, 154
  carbohydrates and, 237
Turmeric, 199–200
Turnip greens, 19
Turnips, phytochemicals in, 295

U
Udon noodles, 251
Ugly fruits, 21

V
Vegetable broth, 115
Vegetable juices, 115, 289
Vegetable oils, heart-healthy,
  113–114
Very-low-density lipoprotein
  (VLDL), 95
Vinegars in low-cholesterol cook-
  ing, 112–113
Vitamin B-12
  deficiencies, 152–153
  miso as source of, 158
Vitamin C
  as antioxidant, 2, 5–7
  in chili peppers, 200

Vitamin C, *continued*
    food sources, 6
    freezing foods and, 6
    in leafy greens, 16
    quick-cooking foods for, 6–7
    vitamin E and, 6
Vitamin E
    as antioxidant, 2, 9–10
    boosting intake of, 10
    food sources, 9–10, 12
    vitamin C and, 6

W

Water, fiber and, 56
Watercress, 119
    phytochemicals in, 295
Wehani rice, 246
Weight loss
    blood pressure and, 192
    cholesterol and, 98
    complex carbohydrates and, 239
West Indian pumpkin, 25
Wheat, 62–63. *See also* Whole
    wheat
Wheat berries, 63
Wheat bran, 63
Wheat germ, 63
White beans, 59
White peppercorns, 198–199
White rice. *See* Rice

White wine, 115
White wine vinegar, 113
Whole foods, advantages of, 13–14
Whole grains
    amino acids in, 155
    complex carbohydrates in, 240,
      246–249
    cooking guide, 247
    fiber from, 52, 55, 60–62
    rice blends, 246
Whole wheat
    couscous, 61–62
    flour, 63
    pasta, 63
    spaghetti, 251
Wild rice, 62, 246
    amino acids in, 155
Wine mustard, 115
Wines in low-cholesterol cooking,
    114–115
Winter squash, 22–25
    tips on, 23

Y

Yogurt, 116
Yukon Gold potatoes, 252

Z

Zeaxanthin, 8, 9, 283, 291

A Note About the Author

JAY SOLOMON has been cooking and writing about food for over a decade. As a chef, teacher, and author of ten cookbooks, Jay brings a wealth of experience to the kitchen and classroom. For many years he owned Jay's Cafe, a healthful, tropical-theme restaurant, and J.J.'s Cookies and Cafe, an upscale gourmet take-out business.

Jay teaches epicurean cooking classes throughout the United States and appears frequently on television talk shows. His articles on food have appeared in a variety of magazines and newspapers, including *The Vegetarian Times*, *Restaurants USA*, and the online edition of the Chicago *Tribune*. Jay graduated from the School of Hotel Administration at Cornell University in 1983. He is currently working on his twelfth cookbook.